My Journey into the World of Intermittent Fasting

Kenneth R. Szulczyk, Ph.D.

I wrote this book as accurately as possible and tried to stick to the known facts about fasting. Although I hold a Doctor of Philosophy (Ph.D.), I am not a medical doctor. I research renewable energy and behavioral finance – i.e., studying the behavior of investors in the financial markets.

Any recommendations and suggestions I have made in this book are for entertainment because fasting constitutes a dangerous activity. A faster with health problems, medical complications, or fasting for an extended time can jeopardize their health and life. Anyone wishing to fast should consult a medical doctor or professional before proceeding. The author or publisher is not liable for readers abusing the information in this book.

The author mentions and refers to many trademarked products in this book. The author does not endorse or receive any financial support for those products.

Table of Contents

Preface

Fasting is a journey with many twists and turns. We may not be exploring ancient stone ruins in the jungles of Cambodia or savoring the exotic flavors of spicy Thai cuisine from the food carts on the streets of Bangkok. However, fasting entails many different methods and strategies, which is why I call it a journey to a healthy body. Fasting has impacted my life profoundly. I did not uncover the fountain of youth. Instead, I discovered a lifestyle to keep my body performing at its best. I feel better and am in better shape at 54 than at 20!

Thus, I had to write a book about fasting because fasting embodies a simple strategy—abstain from food for a time period. It cannot get simpler than that. For example, I researched many types of supplements. I read articles on Chinese medicinal herbs when I shopped at Chinese herbal stores in Malaysia. When I discovered hyaluronic acid, astaxanthin, and lingzhi, I thought I had found three powerful supplements to keep me young, the fountain of youth contained in bottles.

I chose these supplements because of their anti-aging properties. Hyaluronic acid is scattered across the human body and concentrated in the skin, eyes, and joints. Hyaluronic acid, an anti-aging agent, gives people a youthful appearance. Then astaxanthin, a powerful antioxidant, neutralizes free radicals in the body. Free radicals, i.e., charged molecules, harm cells and tissues. One theory of aging blames free radicals as the culprit in aging. At last, lingzhi comes from Chinese and Japanese herbal traditions. Lingzhi, a mushroom that grows on dead trees, is another anti-aging herb; some take lingzhi to treat cancer. People make tea by simmering the dried, sliced mushrooms in water or taking capsules of crushed lingzhi spores.

Then I discovered fasting. If anyone asked me to pick the best antiaging agent, I would choose fasting unequivocally. The herbs and supplements do not come a close second. That idea blows away the mind. We always search for something to add to our diets to make us healthy. Who would have guessed that abstaining from food for a period would awaken powerful repair processes in the body? Of course, humanity has always known this because most of the world's religions advocate fasting. However, our modern society has ignored these ancient religious practices even though it appears we have many sick people walking among us. Modern medicine scoffs at fasting as it sweeps fasting under the rug of superstitious beliefs. Instead, the pharmaceutical companies have every young American hooked on a cornucopia of drugs. Many countries have followed the United States and encouraged the heavy medication of their citizens. Then we see obesity and poor health exploding across the world. I also lived and worked in Malaysia, which is considered the obesity capital of Asia.

I took everything that I knew and read about fasting and compiled it into a book. I look at various sources, including articles from scientific journals, books, and blogs. Although we should be careful of blogs because anyone can write and post blogs online, they provide testimony and information on fasting because the bloggers practice fasting. For example, I found blogs where fasters claimed they excreted dead worms on their fifth day of fasting. Intestinal worms and flora, like yeast, love sugar and carbohydrates. So, a fast starves intestinal parasites. I also examine old references such as Upton Sinclair – *The Fasting Cure* (1911) [1] and the medical doctors Dr. Edward Hooker Dewey (1900) [2] and Herbert Shelton [3]. Dr. Dewey wrote his book in 1900 when he advocated for readers to skip breakfast to improve their health. Dr. Shelton conducted over 30,000 fasts and published the first edition of his book in 1934 [3].

This book provides a wealth of information. I hope people will use it to improve their lives. We can revive one of humanity's ancient practices and restore balance in the world.

1. Introduction

"A genuine fast cleanses the body, mind and soul. It crucifies the flesh and to that extent sets the soul free."

– Mahatma Gandhi

We start the book by explaining the definition of fasting and how fasting differs from starvation. Whenever one mentions fasting, people conjure up an image where they harm themselves by starving or having anorexia. I have seen many blank stares and raised eyebrows when I told people that I couldn't eat because I was fasting. Then we connect fasting to the animal world since all living forms have internal mechanisms to help them survive periods of famine. Finally, we describe the fasting state and what fasters experience.

What is Fasting?

We define fasting as abstaining from all food and drink except water. Water is one of those vital substances we cannot go without for a prolonged period. Although we fast, we should still drink water because water comprises about 60% of an adult man's body, while adult women carry about 55% [4]. We also call this a water fast because fasters are allowed to drink water. The name denotes the type of fast.

The growing popularity of fasting has spawned several variations of fasting that some experts believe are not true fasts. For example, the purists do not accept words like the juice fast because the juice faster does not abstain from the juice—instead, the faster drinks fruit and vegetable juices as part of his or her fasts. Meanwhile, fasters consume beef cooked in a pool of butter as the beef-butter fast. Technically, these are not true fasts since the users consume calories.

The purists reject the notion of the fasting cure. Technically, fasting is a state that allows the body to switch on repair and cleansing processes. Of course, we should not fuss about exact definitions because life is too short. However, we must use precise definitions so we stay on the same page. The word fasting in this book refers to fasting from food and drinks except for water.

Humans fasted since the dawn of civilization. Fasting intertwines with the world's major religions. The three great prophets, Prophet Muhammad, Jesus, and Buddha, fasted. Furthermore, the American Indians and people from ancient Assyria, Egypt, Persia, Babylon, Scythia, Greece, Rome, India, and Palestine practiced fasting as religious rites [3]. Thus, all religions embed fasting.

The following famous biblical characters fasted.

➤ Both Moses and Jesus fasted for 40 days (Exodus 34:28 and Matthew 4:2 [5]).

➤ David fasted for seven days (2 Samuel 12:16 [5]).

➤ The Prophet Elijah fasted for forty days (1 Kings 19:8 [5]).

➤ Esther fasted for three days (Esther 4:16 [5]).

➤ Luke fasted twice a week, which we call intermittent fasting (Luke 18:12 [5]).

➤ Saul, the ruthless prosecutor of early Christians, met the reincarnated Jesus on the way to Damascus. At the site of Jesus, Saul became blind. He abstained from all food and drink for three days and regained his eyesight. Saul transformed into Paul, one of the most influential disciples of Jesus. Paul spread the Christian faith across the Roman Empire (Acts 9:9 [5]).

Various religious groups fast include the following:

➤ Mormons of the Church of Latter-day Saints fast one Sunday out of each month. They practice dry fasting when abstaining from food, drinks, and water.

> ➤ Followers of Judaism practice dry fasting during Yom Kippur, or Day of Atonement, the holiest day of the year.

> ➤ Buddhists claim fasting is meditation for the body. Once monks finishes eating for the day, they can focus on their mental development and meditate for the rest of the day. The Buddhists strive for enlightenment [6].

> ➤ The followers of the Jain religion perform extreme fasting. The Jain religion, an offshoot from Buddhism, was founded in the fourth century, B.C., in northern India [7]. The Jains fast until they starve themselves to death to reach spiritual enlightenment [7].

The early Christians combined prayer and fasting, but the Bible and church, with its numerous denominations, have no doctrine that requires fasting. Christians usually fast during Lent and Advent but few practice in the West. On the other hand, Eastern Orthodox Christians fast regularly during religious holidays.

Muslims are required to fast and abstain from all food and drink between sunrise and sunset during the month of Ramadan as directed by Allah. The Muslims do not have a choice. Muslims also perform the most difficult fast, a dry fast, when they cannot even drink water during the fast. The Prophet Muhammad also advocated that Muslims should fast twice a week on Mondays and Thursdays during all months except Ramadan. Ramadan serves as the annual cleanse, while the twice-weekly fasts serve as maintenance fasts, otherwise known as intermittent fasting.

Buddhism does not have a doctrine for fasting. However, Buddhist monks in China, Tibet, and Thailand practice intermittent fasting. For example, the Thai monks finish their last day's meal at noon and do not eat again until the next morning every day. The Thai monks start breakfast at 8 AM [6, 8]. Thus, they have an eating window of four hours and fast for the remaining 20 hours daily.

Several famous people, such as the three great Greek philosophers Socrates, Plato, and Pythagoras, fasted to boost their brain power and intelligence. Socrates and Plato fasted for 10 days periodically, while Pythagoras fasted for 40 days before taking his entrance examination at the University of Alexandria. Then Pythagoras required his students to fast for 40 days before they could enroll in his class. We see in Chapter 2 that research indicates that fasting boosts brain function. Now, it makes sense to see the connection between fasting and prayer in many religious faiths and why some intellectuals fast. They use fasting to connect to their spirituality.

Political dissidents fast as a political weapon. For example, the national Hindu leader, Gandhi, fasted to gain India's freedom from the British Empire. A doctor monitored Gandhi to ensure he did not endanger his health or life. Gandhi fasted 17 times as a political statement against the British occupation of India, with the longest fast being 21 days [9]. Members of the Irish Republican Army (IRA), such as McSwiney and Joseph Murphy, went on a hunger strike while incarcerated in a British prison. Murphy died after 68 days without food, while McSwiney died in 74 days. Their political fasts failed against the British as the British allowed them to waste away in their jail cells.

A leader imposes a fast upon citizens to unite the country and bring God's favor. The King Jehoshaphat "proclaimed a fast throughout all Judah" as a vast army marched towards the cities of Judah (2 Chronicles 20:2-3 [5]). The king and his people wanted God's attention so God would help Judah defeat its enemies.

Some fasters sought fame and popularity from public fasts because fasting freaks people out. In the 19th century, Succi, Merlatti, and Jacque performed public, extended fasts, and charged admissions fees. They fasted between 21 and 46 days as the audience gawked and watched [3].

People, at last, fast for health reasons. Mother nature has programmed fasting into our bodies. We lose our appetite when we become sick, ill, or injured [9, 10]. When the flu bug strikes, our bodies refuse to keep down food or drink, including water. Thus, our bodies force us into a dry fast. Many times, we go against our bodies' wishes. We have this warped perception that we must eat to maintain our health and strength. Plus, fasting freaks people out. We sabotage ourselves and drink 7-up because we can keep 7-up down while sick.

Thus, the 7-up ends the dry fast because the sugar kicks us out of the fasting state. Since we know the power of fasting while sick, we should only drink 7-up if we feel dehydrated or need that sugary energy. Otherwise, we should fast during sickness.

Fasting versus Starvation

Researchers and scientists often confuse fasting and starvation, which are different processes. Then reporters and journalists provoke public fear when they attribute the dangers or side effects of starvation to fasting.

Dr. Jason Fung defines *fasting* as the voluntary abstaining from food while starvation is involuntary [11, 12]. This definition rings true because people practicing fasting voluntarily abstain from food for a period. However, unfortunate events force some unwilling people into fasting. For instance, sailors shipped wrecked on a deserted island or miners trapped in a collapsed mine were forced into fasting if they had no food or rations [3, 9]. In some cases, the sailors and miners with some food rations were in worse shape than those forced into fasting [3]. The sailors and miners, who had food rations, forced themselves into starvation and not a fasting state. Other unfortunate events force people into fasting, such as famine from drought, crop and cattle failure, floods, tornadoes, earthquakes, snow storms, and wars [3].

As food becomes scarce, people spread their limited food over a day. For example, a person with only 1,000 calories of food will divide the food ration into three meals during the day. In this case, the person keeps the body starving because the periodic feeding hampers and halts the fasting state. If that same person eats all 1,000 calories in one meal, then the person begins fasting 12 hours later. One meal a day is close to a 24-hour fast. The fasting state causes the body to burn fat reserves. Once the faster has depleted their fat reserves, they enter starvation [9]. The body has no other tissues to break down into energy except vital tissues and muscles.

Fasting and starvation impact the organs in the human body differently. Fasting first uses the least vital tissues, such as stored fat [3]. For example, fasting consumes 97% of the body fat in terms of weight, while the spleen loses 67%, the liver 54%, and the testes 40% [3]. The liver loses weight from losing glycogen and water [3, 13]. Glycogen is stored sugar in the liver and muscles. At last, the nervous system and heart lose the least weight, about 3% [3]. On the other hand, starvation consumes the body's critical tissues and organs and jeopardizes the person's life [3, 9]. Then starvation causes a person's core body temperature to drop as the body scrambles to conserve all energy [14].

Fasting Ensures Life's Survival

Biologists define two life cycles: Anabolic and catabolic [3]. Living organisms build structures during the anabolic phase and break down complex structures into simple ones to release energy during the catabolic phase. We refer to the two cycles simply as feasting and fasting.

Fasting is a part of the cycle of life because all lifeforms alternate between periods of feasting and fasting. Feasting supplies the body with nutrients to build structures while fasting performs the house cleaning and maintenance of the body. Somewhere in our history, we have forgotten fasting. Even in 1911, Upton Sinclair wrote about how doctors objected to fasting [1], and we still witness this hostility towards fasting today. Everyone in the modern world clings to feasting while they neglect fasting. Then the healthcare industry is powerless to prevent or cure heart disease, diabetes, and obesity.

Many animals switch between feasting and fasting. For example, animals and insects build body structures during spring and summer and hibernate during late fall and winter. During hibernation, the bears, gophers, chipmunks, and squirrels fast as they survive on their fat deposits. During warm winter days, bears may come out of hibernation to search for food, while squirrels awaken and consume some of their stored nuts [3]. Finally, queen bees burrow into a hole in the ground while wasps hibernate in loose bark on dead trees [3]. They can survive winter on their stored energy.

Tropical countries alternate between wet and dry seasons. Accordingly, animals, insects, and reptiles become dormant during dry seasons in tropical climates as food becomes scarce. Fish, crocodiles, and frogs burrow themselves in the mud as the dry season starts, a process called aestivating. The mud hardens while the fish and reptiles go dormant while entombed in the dirt. At the beginning of the wet season, the torrential rains soften the mud; then the creatures exit their dens as food becomes plentiful again [3].

All species of life have fasting built in. Cats, dogs, cows, horses, deer, and other animals fast when injured or sick [3, 9, 14]. Dr. Shelton provided many examples of injured dogs that fasted to cure themselves [3]. For example, one dog was hit by a truck and suffered multiple broken bones and internal injuries. Another dog accidentally ate rat poison, while a third lost an eye to a cat. The dogs abstained from food for three weeks and survived their injuries.

Cats, to their owners' annoyance, will hide if sick or injured. For example, I gave my cats deworm medication because two of the cats displayed symptoms of worms – a bloated, inflated abdomen and one cat had poop covered with white specks. The two cats abstained from food for two days to allow their digestive system to heal. Then they lost that pudgy look and became slender and active. Please refer to Dr. Shelton's book for more examples and stories on animal fasting [3].

We also provide tips on fasting for animals.

> **Tip #1:** Do not fast your kitties. A cat's liver cannot process large amounts of fats during fasting or starvation because the liver becomes swollen, yellow, and fatty [15]. A cat will die if the liver shuts down. Thus, I feed my kitties twice daily, at 6 AM and 6 PM. Furthermore, they have one hour to eat all the food they want. If we keep refilling the food dish, the cats become periodic snackers, returning every several hours to snack. Then they gain weight. Thus, the strict feeding regimen keeps kitties slender, active, and naughty. We must research the nutritional needs of other animals.

Humans, similar to animals, can survive without food for extended periods because we carry vast stores of fat. For example, a man weighing 200 pounds (90.9 kg) with a body mass index of 25% stores about 50 pounds (22.7kg) of fat. One pound of fat consists of

3,500 calories, and a person usually loses one pound per day on a fast [3]. Therefore, a man could survive 50 days of fasting because the body has plenty of fat reserves to power the body. Most likely, a man will experience health problems when the fat reserves drop below 10% of the body mass index, which gives the man 30 days of fasting. Thus, the human body can survive without food for extended periods.

Fasting is built into the body as if by intelligent design [3]. The body consumes tissue and internal reserves by the ease of rebuilding them when food becomes available again. After the body processes the last meal, the body begins utilizing glycogen from the liver. As glycogen reserves start dropping, the body starts making glucose via gluconeogenesis and switching to burning fat. The body depletes fat reserves and consumes nonvital tissues, such as muscle. Of course, the body conserves the critical organs for last, such as the brain, heart, and lungs [3].

The Fasting State

The body needs time to transition from the feeding state to the fasting state. After we have eaten our last meal, our digestive system takes between three and five hours to process that meal [10]. Hence, the meal provides energy and powers our bodies. After our digestive system has processed the meal, our bodies switch to burning the stored glucose, called glycogen. The liver holds between 80 and 125 grams of glycogen, which equals between 400 and 500 calories of energy [9, 16], while the muscles store between 1,400 and 2,000 calories. An average, moderately active male needs about 2,800 calories daily, while a woman needs about 2,000. After 24 hours, the liver loses about 57% of its glycogen in healthy young males [13].

After we enter a fasting state, our bodies switch from burning glucose, i.e., sugar, and begin burning fat. Experts believe we enter a fasting state between 8 and 12 hours after the last meal [10], but it depends on the person and their activity. (It sounds like the body scrambles to search for nutrients even though the liver has lost about 29% of its glycogen [13]). Subsequently, a person's insulin level starts dropping. Of course, we can use one trick to enter the fasting state sooner, which leads to the second tip.

> ➢ **Tip #2**: Exercise allows fasters to enter the fasting state sooner. We should do aerobic exercise within five hours after eating our last meal. Aerobic exercise depletes the stored glycogen in the muscles. For example, I run on the elliptical trainer for 45 minutes and burn between 400 and 500 calories. Aerobic exercise also imparts many health benefits that complement the health benefits of fasting.

The body enters ketosis between one and three days after beginning the fast [9, 11]. Lean individuals enter ketosis quicker than the obese [17], which seems quite unfair. In addition, women enter ketosis quicker than men [9, 17] and experience quicker drops in blood glucose [17]. Unfortunately, the timing does not add since fasters feel the effects of fasting after eight hours after the last meal. Where does the body get its energy? Do not worry; we will answer this question later.

During ketosis, our body taps into fat stores while the liver metabolizes the fat into ketones. The liver breaks down the fat, or triglyceride, into three molecules of fatty acids and one molecule of glycerol [11, 17]. The 'tri' in triglyceride refers to the three fatty acid molecules. Then the liver converts these fatty acids into ketones – acetoacetate and beta-hydroxybutyrate, which most cells in the body use as energy and create acetone as a waste byproduct [3, 18, 19]. For example, during a fast, people experience a four- to six-fold increase in ketones compared to their feasting day [20]. The body's cells improve the conversion of ketones into energy as opposed to sugar [18]. The presence of ketones could also be the mechanism that suppresses appetite [21]. Lean people may have higher beta-hydroxybutyrate concentrations in the blood than the obese for a 72-hour fast [22]. It is worth noting that most cells in the body can burn fatty acids directly, except the brain and red blood cells.

Several body cells, such as the liver and red blood cells, still burn glucose for energy [9, 17]. Furthermore, the brain requires up to 25% of glucose, with ketones supplying the rest [11]. We need not worry about the absence of sugar because the liver manufactures glucose from amino acids or glycerol using a process called gluconeogenesis [3, 11, 17, 19]. Gluconeogenesis stands for glucose in gluco, neo for new, and genesis for creation [11]. During fasting, the body breaks down muscle into amino acids, or the body breaks down fat, i.e., triglycerides into fatty acids and glycerol [11, 17]. Then the liver manufacturers both glycerol and amino acids into glucose. At last, gluconeogenesis consumes energy, which helps explain why fasters experience a boost in metabolism [23].

Amino acids are the building blocks of proteins. Our bodies require nine amino acids: Histidine, isoleucine, leucine, lysine, methionine, phenylalanine, threonine, tryptophan, and valine. Here is the beauty of fasting. Fasting places the body into scavenger mode as it searches the body for amino acids. One source of proteins is muscles. Several studies show a loss of muscle mass during fasts [9, 23, 24]. Muscle wasting slows after two or three days, which is called muscle-sparing [9, 17]. Autophagy and programmed cell death also supply amino acids, which we discuss in Chapters 2 and 3. Then the body switches to ketones as its fuel source.

Several other factors induce ketosis other than fasting, such as intense, prolonged exercise, low-carbohydrate diets, alcoholism, and starvation.

Some people confuse ketosis and ketoacidosis. People with Type 1 diabetes can suffer from the dangerous condition of ketoacidosis, when both the glucose and ketones rise significantly in the blood at the same time and turn the blood into acid. The immune system of Type I diabetics attacks their pancreas, so the pancreas no longer produces insulin, and the absence of insulin cannot reduce sugar blood levels. The cells have an insulin receptor that allows glucose to enter. In addition, alcoholics starve their bodies of glucose in the presence of alcohol, which could lead to ketoacidosis.

The body possesses powerful control systems to prevent ketoacidosis. Ketones do not elicit an insulin response without glucose [25]. However, in the presence of glucose, ketones, especially beta-hydroxybutyrate, amplify the insulin response in mice [25] and dogs [26]. Then the insulin messages the cells to utilize glucose for energy, and the fat cells store sugar and stop releasing fat. Thus, ketones and blood glucose would never be high simultaneously for people with a normally functioning pancreas.

Some dieters purchase various devices to measure ketones because of the popularity of the ketogenic diet, a diet high in fat and low in carbohydrates. Fasters may also use these devices to measure the degree of ketosis in their bodies and the strength of the fast. The measures include:

- ➤ **Ketosis Test Strips:** People can buy these strips over the counter in any pharmacy for about $10 for 50 sticks—the strips test for acetoacetate. People urinate on the stick for two seconds, shake the stick, and wait 15 seconds for the stick to change color. The sticks pose two problems; once a faster adapts to burning fat, that person may stop excreting acetoacetate, which the test strips check. The body conserves resources efficiently and minimizes acetoacetate excretion [16]. In addition, excessive water drinking and dehydration may cause inaccurate ketone readings.

- ➤ **Electronic Keto Breath:** The faster breathes into the device while the machine determines the level of acetone in the breath. The body produces acetone as a waste product. The machines range between $50 and $100.

- ➤ **Blood Ketone Meter:** These machines are similar to glucose meters, where people with diabetes prick their fingers and measure their blood glucose. The machines are inexpensive, around $30. However, the ketone test strips cost about $1 each. Ouch! The meter tests for the ketone, beta-hydroxybutyrate. We discuss this ketone further in this book because it signals the body's cells to regenerate.

The key ketone is beta-hydroxybutyrate. One study concluded that urine and keto breath correlate with beta-hydroxybutyrate in the blood [27]. However, the study relied on a 12-hour fast followed by a day on the ketogenic diet [27]. The study's limitation is that the researchers did not check for the body's adaption to the fasting state and whether the acetone in the keto breath remains a reliable indicator of beta-hydroxybutyrate.

Once the fasters or dieters have tested their ketone level, they compare the ketone level to Table 1 to indicate the strength of the fast. A strong fast means a person's body is burning more fats. People in good health should never exceed 4.0. Fasting beyond 3 days may raise beta-hydroxybutyrate around 6.0 [19], indicating a strong state of ketosis. Any readings above 8.0 indicate strong ketosis and possible ketoacidosis. Ketoacidosis requires a high blood sugar level while the blood becomes more acidic. Thus, we rush to the hospital as fast as we can.

Table 1. Ketone Levels

Activity	Ketosis Strength	Range (mM / L)
Sugar burner	Zero	0.0
12 – 16 hours fasting	Trace	0.5
Two-day fast	Small	1.0 – 2.0
90 minutes intense exercise	Small	1.0 – 2.0
Ketogenic diet	Small	2.0
Fasting beyond 3 days	Moderate	4.0
Call an ambulance immediately	Large	8.0

Note: The machines and test strips measure ketones by the milli-mole per liter, or mM / L. In chemistry, a mole represents 6.02×10^{23} molecules. We can convert mM / L into milli-grams per deci-liter by multiplying by 10. A deciliter equals 0.1 liters.

I have fasted twice weekly for at least 24 hours per fast for four years. After I fast for 24 hours, the urine keto sticks indicate zero ketones. However, my body begins excreting acetoacetate once I fast beyond 30 hours. I also noticed that if I eat two high-fat, low-carb meals before the fast, jog for at least 30 minutes while fasting, or do both, the keto sticks detect ketosis sooner. According to the urine test strips, the strongest state of ketosis I have experienced was a 4, but I had never fasted beyond two days.

We must remember that urine ketone sticks may not be accurate. The blood ketone meter is the best option if fasters want an accurate measure of ketosis's strength.

***

We switch our attention and discuss what the fasting state feels like. Fasting resembles exercise. We feel the strain and pain the first mile (or kilometer) we run. The sweat burns our eyes while the joints and muscles creak and ache. Then we return home and collapse on the bed. Then each time we run, we become stronger, faster, and healthier. The pain subsides. The body recovers quickly while each mile (or kilometer) becomes easier. Then we run 6.7 miles (10 kilometers) with ease in no time.

Fasting resembles exercise. The more fasts we perform, the easier it is for us to abstain from food and drink. Do not get me wrong. I thought I would die when I did my first 18-hour fast. I felt awful and weak, and I became dizzy after standing up. After each fast, the process became easier and more comfortable. After four years of fasting, I have few difficulties entering a fasting state, as fasting has become second nature.

When I started fasting, I needed a crutch to survive. So, eight hours after my last meal, I ate two hard-boiled eggs with hot sauce. Technically, I violated the fast by eating the eggs, but I needed a little help to get me through. Once the fasts became easy, I no longer needed a crutch.

> **Tip #3:** We use a crutch to help our bodies adjust to fasting. We eat a high-fat, high-protein snack or add a little milk or cream to our coffee and tea. The ketogenic diet also offers many low-carbohydrate snacks. The keto ice cream and chocolate nut clusters are fantastic.

I could sense when I was entering a fasting state. A euphoria and peacefulness swept across my mind after eight hours after my last meal. My senses sharpened and became more sensitive. Colors were brighter, while sounds and smells became stronger. I enjoyed riding my motorcycle at dusk, watching the vibrant Borneo sunsets, or watching a movie with friends at the cinema. I am a young kid again, jolting and screeching during the scary parts of a good movie. If I fast during the day, I must wear sunglasses as the bright, intense sun rays blast down upon me.

> ➤ **Tip #4:** Most fasters experience the fasting euphoria. If we experience euphoria, we should enjoy it, such as watching a good film or connecting with nature by gardening, hiking, or taking the kids or pets to the park. We can let the rolling ocean waves soothe us as we stroll along the beach. Fasting connects us with nature and unplugs us from the modern world for a while.

The euphoria comes from the adrenaline our bodies produce when entering the fat-burning state—no wonder many religions incorporate fasting. Fasting is spiritual and awakens an inner peacefulness.

When we begin fasting, we must be careful the first several times. For instance, the euphoria makes some people spacey. Several times, I almost turned in front of oncoming traffic on my motorcycle. Furthermore, we should avoid exercising during the first few fasts. However, we can return to our exercise regimens once fasting becomes second nature. I experienced no problems doing my resistance training or running on fasting days. Running intensifies the water fast as I deplete and burn the sugar in my body.

A faster will notice several things to indicate that he or she is fasting. After eight hours into the fast, we should smell ketones on our breaths. We call this the Adkin's or Keto breath after the Adkin's or Keto Diets because the low carbohydrate diet triggers ketosis and the associated bad breath. As the body metabolizes ketones for energy, the body produces acetone as a waste product. The body expels acetone in the breath and urine, giving faster that nasty, foul-smelling breath. The ketones also suppress appetite and hunger pangs [21].

During a fast, a white coating covers the tongue. Dr. Shelton, Dr. Weber, and the writer Upton Sinclair claimed that a white tongue indicated that the body was expelling toxins [1-3]. We can debate this notion. Some contended that fasters experienced bacteria and yeast overgrowth in the mouth during a fast. That is illogical because these organisms crave sugar, and the body has already metabolized the sugar. Thus, the yeast and bacteria should die from the lack of food. Logically, the food acts like sandpaper on the tongue, especially the tortilla and potato chips. When the faster the stops eating food, the tongue keeps producing cells that coat the tongue's surface. Thus, the tongue turns white as a faster abstains from abrasive food.

Dr. Dewey, Dr. Shelton, and Mr. Sinclair used the tongue as an indicator [1-3, 14]. When the tongue had returned to its normal color, the faster's hunger had returned, or both, the person ended the fast [1-3, 14, 28]. Dr. Shelton and Sinclair performed extended fasts of two weeks or more [1, 3], while Dr. Dewey skipped breakfast daily except to enjoy his morning cup of coffee [2]. However, waiting for the tongue to return to normal color may be an unreliable indicator.

Fasters will notice other signs, such as the disappearance of allergies. For example, I am allergic to tree pollen. Unfortunately, the Year 2018 was my worst year for allergies because I lived in Borneo, Malaysia, where a tree bloomed every several months. However, my sinuses and nose cleared after abstaining from food for eight hours. The redness of my eyes faded; I still sneezed occasionally, but I could sit under the offending tree without ill effect. The culprit is the body producing histamines to combat the pollen.

Other fasting effects include the following:

> **Constipation**: No food coming in means nothing going out [9, 11, 14]. Some fasters mention they still have healthy bowel movements during the fast. During the early 20th century, doctors performed enemas on fasters because the doctors thought the stools would solidify into a rock or the body's colon would assimilate decaying waste [1, 3, 14, 28, 29]. Although these fasts extend beyond two weeks, we can debate whether we need enemas.

Some fasters claimed they excreted dead worms and parasites from five-day fasts. Intestinal worms and parasites crave sugar, so fasting eliminates their food source. What is odd is that scientists have fasted worms in the laboratory. Those little critters still survive after consuming most of their body during a fast. Thus, the critters can fast, too, which extends their lives.

> **Dark Urine:** Some fasters report dark urine, while others describe black sediment in their urine during extended fasts. Of course, fasting cleanses and detoxifies the body. During the feasting cycle, the body sweeps the dust and debris under the rug to eliminate it. The body usually tucks toxins into the fatty tissue. Subsequently, fasting burns the fat and releases the toxins into the body again. Then the body must rid itself of these toxins during a fast, such as the urine.

> **Headaches:** Some fasters experience headaches. The headaches may result from the body ridding itself of toxins or the faster has abstained from caffeine.

> **Metabolism**: Fasting boosts metabolism [23], or at least it does not slow it down for fasts with durations less than 36 hours [30].

> **Periods of Weakness:** Fasters alternate between high energy and weakness periods. For example, I usually have energy during a fast. However, I occasionally feel weak and sluggish during a fast. The temporary weakness goes away. Please note that if we feel terrible during a fast, we should eat something to break the fast. Our health comes first, then the duration of a fast. We can always live another day and fast at another time.

> **Insomnia** [9, 14, 29]: Some fasters sleep better while other fasters sleep around four hours [14] and report disturbances in their sleep [31]. Unfortunately, I experience sleeping problems during extended fasts. I often sleep four hours while fasting

rather than my usual eight hours. However, I still function normally throughout the day on partial sleep.

➢ **Feeling Cold**: The faster feels cold because the body conserves energy during a fast [9, 29]. The faster should dress warmly and wrap in a blanket for warmth.

➢ **Blurry Vision**: Some fasters experience blurry vision or have trouble focusing their eyes [29].

➢ **Hair and Fingernails**: The hair softens in texture [3]. Meanwhile, a faster experiences slower hair and fingernail growth, especially during extended fasts [3]. Some fasters experience hair loss during extended fasts [29]. The body prioritizes its energy consumption when the energy source, i.e., food, becomes scarce. The body assigns hair and fingernail growth as low priorities.

Of course, the best part of the fast is breaking the fast. Our taste buds are sensitive. Our digestive system has rested and roars to process food again. When we take that first bite, taste sensations tickle our tongues. The food is delicious. That is why I appreciate the engineering and creativity of corporations designing our food. I broke fasts with a bag of Doritos and a Snickers, a Big Mac with French fries, and pizza, but not at the same time. Thus, a fast allows us to enjoy food during our feasting cycle.

After fasting intermittently for four years, I no longer get the white-coated tongue, smell the ketones on my breath, or experience sensitive senses. My taste buds lack sensitivity when I break a fast. Now, I feel little difference between fasting and feasting. Usually, I must fast beyond 30 hours to experience the faster's euphoria. However, I am not a junky chasing after my first high. I define clearly why I fast; I fast to get the health benefits. I do not extend my fasting time to capture these secondary benefits. Health and safety come first.

2. Health Benefits of Fasting

"Fasting is no cunning trick of priestcraft, but the most powerful and safest of all medicines."

– M. L. Holbrook, a Hygienist

Many diseases originate from chronic inflammation. Inflammation is a natural part of the immune system as white blood cells hunt down and destroy foreign invaders like bacteria and viruses. As we age, cells become damaged and begin releasing chemical messengers called cytokines that cause the immune system to go into overdrive, leading to chronic inflammation. Chronic inflammation harms our cells, organs, and tissues and triggers many diseases as the immune system attacks the body. A group of Japanese researchers believe low levels of inflammation were responsible for the long life of centenarians [32].

Fasting reduces inflammation [33], curing many diseases. Upton Sinclair and Dr. Shelton claimed fasting cures all human ailments except tuberculosis [1, 3]. Upton Sinclair was a prolific American writer at the turn of the 20th while Dr. Shelton supervised over 30,000 fasts [3, 14]. Although Dr. Dewey does not mention tuberculosis, he encouraged intermittent fasting to cure various illnesses. Tuberculosis differs from other illnesses. It is a nasty bacterial infection attacking the lungs and can easily spread from one victim to the next through sneezing, coughing, or talking.

As we will see, fasting impacts the body profoundly. Fasting gives the body a rest from the feasting cycle and allows it to cleanse and repair itself.

Autoimmune Diseases

Fasting helps reduce the problems of autoimmune diseases. The immune system searches the body for foreign material, such as bacteria and viruses. Sometimes, the immune system makes a mistake and attacks healthy cells and tissues instead, which we call autoimmune disease [9]. The disease depends on which tissues and cells the immune system attacks.

The antibodies identify the foreign substances in the body called antigens [9]. The antibodies mistake the body's cells if the cells become too polluted or abnormal [9]. Then the antibodies attach themselves to those abnormal cells and form an antigen-antibody complex [9]. The antigen-antibody complexes can lodge themselves in the tissue and trigger inflammation [9]. For example, people suffering from rheumatoid arthritis experience redness, stiffness, and joint pain as the antigen-antibody complexes build up and create chronic joint inflammation [9].

Fasting is one of the strongest agents to combat inflammation [9, 33]. Thus, fasting reduces the impact of autoimmune diseases quickly [9, 34]. Fasting provides three effects on the body. First, fasting gives the digestive system a rest and allows the digestive system to heal itself [9, 14]. That way, food and foreign substances do not enter the bloodstream. The food leaking into the bloodstream forms antigens that swing the immune system into overdrive [9]. Second, the joints heal as they receive more oxygen and nutrients because the joints rely on the joint fluid to transport nutrients and oxygen [9]. Hence, fasting increases joint circulation [9]. Finally, fasting helps the body clear the antibody-antigen complexes and reduces inflammation during and after a fast [9].

Some people report that fasting cures the following ailments.

> **Multiple Sclerosis** [9, 14, 35]: The immune system attacks and destroys the myelin sheath that covers the nerve cells [9, 36]. The sheath forms insulation around the nerve, like insulation covering wires in a house. The insulation prevents the wires from shorting out and starting a house fire.

> **Grave's Disease**: The immune system attacks the thyroid glands [9].

> **Lupus:** The immune system attacks body tissues and organs [9, 34]. This disease usually inflicts women because high estrogen levels make women more susceptible [9]. Lupus affects the joints, skin, and kidneys and gives sick women a rounded appearance [9].

> **Psoriasis:** The immune system attacks the skin, forming white scales on the skin's surface [9].

> **Rheumatoid Arthritis:** The immune system attacks the joints [9, 36]. Fasting reduces pain and stiffness, so patients reduce medications [34, 35, 37].

Autophagy

Autophagy comes from the word auto, meaning self, and phagein, which means to eat [11]. The word paired together literally means "to eat oneself" [11]. This concept sounds gruesome, but the body needs autophagy to maintain its best health. Autophagy is the process of breaking down damaged and worn-out parts within a cell and recycling the components [11, 38-42]. Autophagy also ensures that cells survive periods of starvation [40, 41]. Then a cell uses the recycled parts to rebuild new structures in the cell [11, 41]. Thus, we are remodeling the kitchen to make it new, sleek, and modern even though we live in an old house.

Autophagy depends on a pathway called the mammalian target of rapamycin, or mTOR for short [11, 40, 41, 43-48]. Every cell in the body possesses the mTOR. We view mTOR as a sensor for insulin, amino acids, oxygen, and energy levels. Thus, as we eat carbohydrates or proteins, the mTOR detects that the body is processing food. Thus, mTOR signals the cells that the body has a supply of nutrients because the body breaks down carbohydrates into glucose which triggers insulin secretion. Meanwhile, the digestive system breaks proteins down into amino acids, thus triggering the mTOR sensor. The presence of mTOR turns off autophagy because the body uses the nutrients to build structures.

When a person fasts, insulin levels drop [17, 48-51] while glucagon rises [17, 50, 51]. Insulin and glucagon are adversaries. Glucagon signals the muscles to release their glycogen or stored sugar. Since the body has no incoming nutrients, mTOR goes dormant and switches on autophagy. Glucagon may also help switch on autophagy by depleting the amino acids [40]. Consequently, the body goes into recycling mode.

The body is incredibly complex, and other conditions can switch on autophagy. For example, when nutrients become scarce, the protein AMPK (adenosine mono-phosphate-activated protein kinase), rises and turns on autophagy directly [41, 42, 45, 47, 48]. AMPK also switches off mTOR [41, 47, 52].

How many hours does a person need to fast for autophagy to turn on? The answers vary from 8 hours to three days, depending on whom we ask. However, we know liver glycogen and insulin drop to low levels after 12 hours into a fast, while glucagon peaks after 13 hours [53]. Our digestive systems would also have processed and assimilated all the protein within this time, so the mTOR should turn off while AMP should switch on, thus activating autophagy.

It is important to recognize that each individual's hormonal response to fasting is unique. A study on overweight participants, for instance, found that the autophagy gene ATG12 was activated during 16-hour fasts [54]. However, it is worth noting that obese individuals and those with diabetes may experience less autophagy [41]. This could be attributed to their elevated and persistently high insulin levels [22], which prevent the inhibition of mTOR and, consequently, the activation of autophagy.

We also cannot measure autophagy since the process occurs within the cells [55]. Some fasters measure their insulin and glucagon levels, or the ratio of insulin to glucagon [56]. Other fasters use ketone strips to measure the level of ketones in their blood or urine. If the body is burning ketones for fuel, then the body should have switched on autophagy. Furthermore, autophagy reacts to stress on a cell, and other pathways switch on autophagy, such as dehydration as in a dry fast, exposure to an extremely hot or cold environment, or hypoxia, i.e., oxygen deprivation. Of course, fasters should not deprive themselves of oxygen.

The mTOR pathway is sensitive, and just 3 grams of leucine, an amino acid, can halt autophagy [11]. Intense exercise also causes mTOR to go dormant and switch on autophagy. In a mice study, 30 minutes of running on a treadmill switched on AMPK and turned off mTOR [57]. Therefore, exercise and autophagy go together like soda and popcorn at the cinema. That is why we fasters must be careful what we drink during a fast. A splash of cream in our coffee may halt autophagy momentarily.

Christian de Duve discovered the process of autophagy and won the Nobel Prize in Physiology and Medicine in 1974. Autophagy depends on lysosomes, a part within every cell. A lysosome acts like a stomach inside a cell and contains digestive enzymes. Subsequently, autophagy causes a lysosome to release the enzymes that digest old, broken-down cell parts, including engulfed bacteria and viruses [41]. Then the cell recycles the parts to build new cell structures [39].

Autophagy comes in three forms.

> **Macroautophagy:** Cells create an autophagosome within a cell. It resembles a tiny Pac-Man that goes around the cell, eating the debris, foreign organisms, and damaged cell structures. The autophagosome engulfs an organelle (or "little organ"), damaged proteins, fats (or lipids), or bacteria in a damaged cell [39, 40, 42-44, 46, 58-60], and then the autophagosome fuses with the lysosome [41-44, 46, 58-61]. The digestive juices of the lysosome break down the damaged organelle into proteins, fatty acids, and raw materials so the body can recycle the components [40, 43]. Furthermore, the cells create autophagosomes during nutrient deficiency or cell stress [44], which are crucial for longevity [45].

Short bouts of fasting can increase the size and number of autophagosomes within cells. In a study of well-fed male mice, scientists detected few and small autophagosomes inside neuron cells or brain cells [62]. After 24 hours of fasting, the autophagosomes multiplied and expanded in size [62]. After 48 hours of fasting, the autophagosomes became larger and became 3 to 4 times as numerous as the well-fed state [62].

Mitophagy and lipophagy are two common forms of macroautophagy. Mitophagy recycles a cell's mitochondria [42, 58, 63], which provide heat and energy to a cell, i.e., the cell's energy furnace. Meanwhile, lipophagy targets autophagy to lipids, i.e., fat.

➢ **Microautophagy:** The lysosome attaches itself directly to the cytoplasm within a cell [42, 44]. The cytoplasm consists of all material in the cell except the nucleus and includes the mitochondria and lipids. Microautophagy does not depend on nutrient deficiency [44]. It is just part of routine maintenance.

➢ **Chaperone-mediated autophagy:** A unique protein selects and binds with material and fuses the material to the lysosome directly [42, 44, 64]. The specific protein scavenges for proteins one by one within a cell. A nutrient deficiency can trigger this selective autophagy [44, 64], which may be critical in a person's longevity [45].

Now, we see why exercise and fasting are essential. Autophagy slows the negative impact of aging and age-related diseases by recycling old parts within a cell [38, 39, 44, 45]. Hence, we take our old, dependable car to a mechanic for a tune-up and some repairs, and that engine purrs like a happy kitten.

We know fasting promotes and stimulates autophagy. Researchers believe the rise of ketones, particularly beta-hydroxybutyrate, messages the body's cells to switch on autophagy [64-66]. We can implement several methods to strengthen autophagy and the state of ketosis during a fast.

1. We exercise during a fast to strengthen autophagy. Both aerobic and resistance training encourage autophagy.

2. We should drink coffee during a fast. Researchers found that regular and decaffeinated coffee encourages autophagy in mice's heart, liver, and muscle cells by raising AMPK and lowering mTOR [59].

3. During a fast, we can drink green tea containing a polyphenol, epigallocatechin gallate (EGCG). In mice, the EGCG turns on AMPK and autophagy in the liver cells [67].

4. Sweating in saunas and shivering in ice baths could spur autophagy because autophagy strengthens the body's cells against external stress. The Russians are on to something as they sit in a hot sauna, then run and jump into an icy lake during winter. They are shocking the body from one extreme to the next extreme and switching on that autophagy. Moreover, we thought the Russians were crazy.

5. The dry fast is the strongest. Refer to Chapter 5 and the fasting types. As the faster deprives himself or herself of nutrients and fluids, the blood concentrates salts like sodium, which causes water to flow out of the cells, a process called hypertonic stress. The cells shrink and switch on autophagy. A cell has microtubules that crisscross the cell like I-beams in a building to maintain the structure and shape. Autophagy switches on to reorganize the microtubules [68]. Researchers need to find out which mechanisms of autophagy are responsible for this reorganization [68].

We can also include several methods to enhance autophagy during our feasting cycle. The ketogenic diet, coconut oil (or medium-chain triglycerides), and supplements such as berberine and resveratrol help promote autophagy by activating AMPK [65, 69].

Bacteria, Viruses, and COVID-19

Fasting rejuvenates and restores the body and immune system as it clears the body of old, poorly working cells and improves the faster's health. Furthermore, autophagy can create autophagosomes that devour bacteria and viruses within the cell and fuse them with a lysosome to break them down into simple proteins. Thus, autophagy kills bacteria and viruses and helps the body rid itself of foreign invaders [43].

The autophagy theory suggests fasting should clear the cells of bacteria and viruses, but the role of fasting is more complicated. We have that old adage – "starve a fever and stuff a cold." For example, fasting may be effective against bacterial infections. In an experiment, fasted mice survived against sepsis and listeria infections, while fed mice succumbed to the bacterial infections [70]. There are two possible mechanisms. Fasting switches the body's fuel from glucose to ketones which limit a bacteria's food source [70]. Bacteria love sugar the same as humans. Furthermore, fasting puts the cells into protection mode and helps them better survive an immune system attack [70]. (We will see this in chemotherapy for cancer).

The role of fasting with viruses is different. Referring to the same experiment, fasted mice died from the influenza virus while the fed mice survived [70] because viruses do not need sugar to survive. They enter a cell, hijack its protein-creating machinery, and start replicating copies of itself. That is why scientists debate whether viruses are alive; they depend on cells for reproduction. The fasted mice succumb to the influenza virus because fasting puts the cells into protection mode. However, the immune system may prefer to destroy the whole infected cell using apoptosis [70]. Apoptosis is when the cell goes through a procedure to destroy itself. The immune system can trigger apoptosis by causing the cell to implode and release its components, including the viruses. There is no cell – thus, no way the virus can replicate. However, more viruses are circulating and can find their way to new cells to replicate.

That brings us to the coronavirus, also known as COVID-19. Between 2020 and 2022, the coronavirus caused a worldwide pandemic that shut down most economies and killed over 6 million people. The victims of COVID-19 shared common comorbidities, which are.

> **Obesity:** Obese people suffer from higher blood glucose levels. They also may have Type 2 diabetes, high blood pressure, chronic inflammation, a weakened immune system, and metabolic dysfunction [71].

> **Diabetes** [72-74]**:** We are referring to Type II diabetes, where the sufferers have chronically high blood sugar levels. These people suffer from a range of diseases known as metabolic

syndrome, including heart disease, high blood pressure, stroke, high cholesterol levels, and obesity.

> **The Elderly:** People aged 65 and older are susceptible to the coronavirus [72-76]. The older we get, the more likely our immune system will not work at peak efficiency, and we will be more susceptible to diseases and infections.

> **Smokers:** Former and current cigarette smokers are susceptible to the coronavirus [72, 76]. Smoking weakens the lungs and serves as an entry point for the virus.

> **Cancer:** Cancer patients are susceptible to the coronavirus [72, 73].

> **Males:** The virus is just being unfair. Men are more likely to die from the coronavirus than women [76].

Does fasting help cure the coronavirus? No research shows that fasting helps shorten or improve the symptoms of COVID-19. However, regular fasting better equips people to fight viral infections because fasting lowers inflammation, blood sugar levels, and obesity and improves health [71, 77, 78]. Thus, fasting reduces most of the risk factors.

A person's blood sugar level indicates how severe someone will suffer from the coronavirus. People with high blood levels are more likely to suffer from complications, be admitted to the intensive care unit, or die from the coronavirus [71, 79]. High blood sugar does the same for the influenza A (H1N1) virus [80], regardless of whether a person has diabetes. High blood sugar levels slow healing and weaken the immune system. Obese people may also develop a weaker immune response to vaccines [71].

Lowering inflammation is an important key for the coronavirus since the coronavirus may cause an inflammatory cytokine storm [81]. The infected cells send out cytokine messengers, i.e., proteins that message the immune system to seek and destroy the threat [33]. However, a cytokine storm is when the cells send out too many messengers, and the immune system goes into hyperdrive, which damages cells and organs. It is like a group of naughty, truant kids lighting fireworks in a neighborhood. All the residents freak out and report gunshots to the police, who send in an army to destroy the neighborhood.

***

Fasting works. I've witnessed an improvement in my health. In 2017, I experienced my worst year. I frequently scuba-dived and passed my rescue diver certification in July 2017. Like clockwork, I would get an ear infection every two months in my right ear, and the virus would take a week or two to go away. My doctor prescribed an ear ointment, but the medicine did nothing. The ear infection returned for a day during the first several fasts and disappeared rapidly. Now, the ear infection has become a fading memory. Dr. Moser called this retracing as fasters relive past infections [29]. I refer to it as a ghost infection. Of course, some fasters experience ghost pains as they relive pain and discomfort from old injuries during a fast.

In November 2017, I caught this nasty respiratory illness with a sore throat, phlegmy rough cough, and fever. Several times, I almost passed out from a coughing fit that lasted a minute. The sickness took two weeks to go away. Then I started my divemaster training in December 2017 in Kota Kinabalu, Malaysia, and the illness returned with a vengeance. I had to take a five-day break to rest and recover from the illness. I finished my divemaster training, but the illness returned with me when I returned home. When I visited a college friend in Bangkok in January 2018, the sickness returned for the fourth time. I could not shake this illness. It was like walking through a field of prickers while hundreds of prickers clinging to my clothes that I could not shake off. When I was young, I rarely got sick; if I did, I recovered in a day or two.

I started intermittent fasting in April 2018, and that illness returned in August and again in December. However, this time was different. I shrugged the virus off like a dog shaking off a flea. I was slightly ill for two days as my body squashed the infection quickly. That leads to a good tip on fasting.

> **Tip #5:** We should start a fast when we feel the onset of a cold, flu, or other illness. Fasting switches the body into repair mode and speeds recovery as the body searches for viruses and bacteria to break down and recycle. I even fasted during two episodes of the coronavirus without any problems.

Brain Function

Intermittent fasting impacts brain function and brain structure profoundly. Both exercise and fasting boost a protein called brain-derived neurotrophic factor (BDNF) [11, 37, 54, 82-84]. BDNF helps the brain's neurons survive injuries and diseases and encourages the growth of new neurons and synapses and, thus, becomes the brain's superfood [37, 83]. A neuron or nerve cell communicates information through electrical impulses, while a synapse forms a junction between two brain cells. The synapse either passes or blocks an electrical signal. The BDNF is vital for brain health and influences higher thinking, learning, and long-term memory.

As people age, their brains degrade and deteriorate over time. For instance, people, usually the elderly, have Alzheimer's Disease, sometimes called Type III diabetes. In the beginning stages of the disease, the victims become forgetful or have trouble thinking [85]. As the disease progresses, the sufferers lose the ability to perform simple tasks [85]. A characteristic of Alzheimer's is the abnormal accumulation of amyloid beta proteins [18, 82, 86]. We view these proteins as toxic garbage and plaques that disrupt the synapses and hamper the communication between neurons in the brain [11, 85, 86]. Researchers believe autophagy stops working or slows down in Alzheimer's patients [85, 87]. Then the amyloid beta proteins accumulate and hamper the electrical signals within the brain.

The good news is that fasting helps people with Alzheimer's because autophagy creates autophagosomes that absorb the amyloid beta proteins and recycle the proteins [11, 85]. A cell under stress creates autophagosomes that gobble the amyloid beta proteins and fuse with a lysosome. The lysosome releases the digestive enzymes that break down the toxic proteins into raw building blocks, amino acids. Furthermore, ketones protect the neurons from death as the cells utilize ketones for fuel [18, 65, 82].

Fasting aids in two additional degenerative brain diseases: Huntington's and Parkinson's. Parents pass Huntington's disease to offspring through their genes. Huntington's disease means the brain cells die over time. The disease starts with mood and thinking problems and progresses to the inability to walk and talk. Like Alzheimer's disease, scientists believe autophagy stops working in the neuron cells because the mTOR becomes defective [87]. In addition, some people inherit Parkinson's disease. The sufferers tend to shake and jerk when they move as the disease affects motor functions. They also have trouble walking. Accordingly, intermittent fasting lessens the symptoms and conditions of Huntington's and Parkinson's diseases [11, 82].

We revert to the mice and rat studies because they age rapidly, and scientists can dissect and examine the rodent's brains under a microscope. In one study, researchers discovered that intermittent fasting boosted rodent memory and learning [88, 89]. Furthermore, the mice's brains showed less oxidative stress than the control group [37, 88]. Oxidative comes from the word oxygen. When oxygen reacts with another chemical, the reaction exchanges electrons. Electrons are negatively charged particles that make electronic devices function. Oxidation is also the chemical reaction of a fire consuming wood and paper, as the fire creates heat and light. The exchange of electrons inside the body causes stress and damage to the cells and tissues. Although our bodies need oxidation to create energy and live, oxidation damages our bodies simultaneously.

In one study, researchers induced strokes in the brains of young, middle-aged, and elderly mice. After intermittent fasting, the young mice had the highest levels of BDNF, while the oldest had the lowest [90]. The youngest and middle-aged fasting mice survived an artificially induced stroke, while the elderly fasting mice were more likely to die from the stroke [90]. The elderly mice had greater concentrations of chemical markers that indicated chronic inflammation [90]. The mice allowed to eat freely with similar age groups resembled the elderly mice that fasted [90]. The well-fed young mice died, too. Consequently, the effects of fasting weaken over time as we age. Otherwise, animals and humans could live forever.

Fasting affects the neurons in the brain. For example, elderly mice genetically prone to Alzheimer's disease exhibited little mental decline for the calorie-restricted and intermittently fasting groups. In contrast, the control group that ate freely showed signs of Alzheimer's disease [86]. Ironically, the calorie-restricted group exhibited less buildup of the amyloid beta proteins in their brains [86]. Although the intermittent fasting and the control groups showed the same level of buildup of the amyloid beta proteins, intermittent fasting strengthened the mice's neurons. It made the neurons more stress-resistant [86]. We must remember that these mice were genetically prone to abnormal protein buildup. Scientists would need to use normal mice to determine whether intermittent fasting removes the protein garbage and plaques from the brain. In another study, fasting mice genetically prone to Huntington's disease showed boosts in BDNF and lived longer with better motor skills than the control group [91].

In another study, rats that fasted intermittently showed boosts in learning, memory, and BDNF [37, 89, 92]. The rats also produced new neurons in the hippocampus [37, 92]. Scientists believe the hippocampus aids in memory storage, motivation, and emotions. In another experiment, fasting rats with spinal injuries recovered quicker than rats that ate freely or were on a calorie-restricted diet [93]. Yes, the scientists deliberately injured the rats' spinal cords as part of the experiment.

Cancer

Cancer occurs when a person's cells mutate and divide uncontrollably. Researchers believe chronic inflammation triggers cancer [94] when it forms abnormal tissues or tumors. The tumors serve no purpose in the human body as they rob the body of nutrients and harm nearby healthy tissues and organs. Cancer can also form from any cell or organ in the body. Unfortunately, the cancerous cells can metastasize and spread to other body parts. For example, skin cancer, which doctors can quickly treat, can spread the cancer to the brain and other vital organs if left untreated.

Normal, healthy cells switch energy sources between glucose and ketones. Our digestive system creates glucose from carbohydrates during our feasting cycle and ketones from fat during our fasting cycle. On the other hand, cancer and tumor cells have a defect or mutation in their energy source. They remain stuck using glucose as their primary energy and cannot switch to ketones. Scientists call this phenomenon the Warburg Effect after the German biochemist Otto Warburg, who discovered this phenomenon in the 1920s [95]. The cancer cells love sugar like children devour their large bulging bags of trick-or-treat candy on Halloween. Thus, we utilize fasting to starve and kill the cancer cells.

We should not be surprised that insulin growth factor and insulin encourage the growth of cancer [96-99]. Insulin signals the body's cells to grow using sugar or glucose, especially cancer cells. Furthermore, the liver produces insulin growth factor that acts like insulin and informs the cells in the body to grow. The insulin growth factor can also prevent apoptosis or programmed cell death. Apoptosis removes the poorly functioning cells that cannot be repaired. In mice, suppressing the insulin growth factor leads to the body creating new cells upon refeeding [100]. Furthermore, people afflicted by obesity or Type 2 diabetes or both have a greater chance of dying from cancer [96, 98, 101].

We can see the importance of fasting. Normal cells switch to ketones, while cancerous cells starve during fasting. For example, a study showed intermittent fasting stifled tumor formation in rats [102] and mice [37, 103, 104]. Participants showed declines in insulin growth factor during short and extended fasts [48, 51, 54, 105, 106]. We expect this because the body switches to conservation and repair mode when no food comes in. Their overall health also improved, which could be a factor.

Rodent studies on fasting show conflicting results because researchers breed specific lines of rodents. Most studies indicate that insulin growth factor stays the same or increases in fasted mice and rats [89, 107], while two studies showed a decrease in insulin growth factor in both mice and rats [97, 108]. Reducing insulin growth factor may be essential to extend longevity and activate longevity genes [42, 109].

For all the rat and mice studies, the fasted rodents experienced the largest drop in blood glucose and insulin [89, 91, 107] and the highest increase in ketones such as beta-hydroxybutyrate [89, 107]. The fasted mice and rats had lower sugar and insulin levels that would slow the growth of cancers despite the higher insulin growth factor. Prolonged fasting also causes cancer cells to transmit fewer chemical markers that hide the cancer from the immune system [99].

Some fasters claimed a complete remission and recovery from cancer [3, 9, 14, 102]. The remission rate of cancer varies with the faster. The body's absorption of a tumor depends on the faster's age and condition, the tumor type, and whether the faster has a hard or soft tumor [3]. Cancer patients must fast for a minimum of 48 hours to inhibit cancer [99], while Dr. Shelton fasted cancer patients for two weeks or more several times to eliminate the cancers [3].

Dr. Joel Fuhrman believes fasting cannot dissolve the tumors of obese people [9]. During a fast, the body devours the most accessible tissues first for energy, which would be the fat stored in obese people. However, we can use one argument to counteract this. Intermittent fasting, diet, and exercise can help an overweight person lose weight. Once the person slims down, fasting helps the body devour the cancer. Intermittent fasting is like cleaning a messy garage. As we clean the garage once or twice a week and only add a little garbage between cleanings, we will open the door one day to a spotless, clean garage. That is the power of intermittent fasting.

Fasting provides another benefit of chemotherapy. Medical doctors use chemotherapy as one of the primary treatments for cancer. The doctors inject a poisonous substance into the body that kills the cancer cells. However, the substance harms and kills healthy cells, tissues, and organs. Consequently, a patient can reduce the adverse side effects of chemotherapy by fasting [37, 38, 99, 103]. Fasting switches the cell's energy source to ketones, which minimizes the impact of chemotherapy because fasting puts the healthy cells into protective mode while the cancer cells are entirely exposed to the poisonous chemicals [99]. One study of mice shows how fasting protects healthy cells and organs but allows poisonous chemotherapy to target and kill cancer cells [37, 103, 110].

We believe the body uses a process called autolysis to remove cancer, unneeded tissues, and cells. Autolysis resembles autophagy, except the cell releases the digestive enzymes from the lysosomes that dissolve the whole cell, while autophagy controls the digestive juices to destroy specific structures within the cell and retain other cell parts. Autolysis originates from Greek and means self-losing [3, 14].

Autolysis is a process observed in various life forms. For instance, if we leave a potato, yam, or onion in a sunny area, life persists. A stem and roots emerge as the plant consumes the bulb or tuber without external nutrients [3]. Another example is the rapid growth of a tadpole, which is facilitated by the tadpole assimilating its tail and using recycled cells to grow legs [3].

Some fasters reported moles, bumps, and scars disappearing after regular bouts of intermittent fasting. I witnessed a dozen bumps and scars disappear after six months of intermittent fasting – some of these bumps I had for ten years or more. Just imagine what fasting does to the inside of our bodies.

We must add a note of caution. Autophagy may weaken the benefits of autolysis. Scientists believe cancer cells utilize autophagy to prolong their life [43, 111, 112]. However, scientists have yet to unravel all the mysteries of autophagy in the body [43]. Perhaps we know the reason why the Soviet doctors would not allow cancer patients to fast [28]. In one study, one day of fasting twice per week did not heal the mice with prostate cancer [113].

The Digestive System

Each time we eat food, we supply the body with energy and nutrients and expose our bodies to additives, artificial coloring, bacteria, and toxins [9]. The body must sort through the food, absorb the nutrients, and dispose of the waste. The body expends about 25% of its energy to break down and process food into energy, making it energy intensive. The immune system also places most of its defenses along the digestive system since it is a major entry point for bacteria and viruses.

Fasting gives the digestive system a rest. The intestines, liver, pancreas, and stomach stop processing food and take a break during a fast. Then the organs heal themselves. For example, a fast improves and repairs the liver. People suffering from alcoholic liver injury, fatty liver, and drug-induced liver damage improve their livers from fasting [9].

Fasting impacts stem cells. Stem cells are blank cells that can become any cell in the body. Stem cells can create new stem cells as needed. The body fashions stem cells to replace broken and damaged cells. Stem cells come in different types, such as stem cells in embryos and adult stem cells. Adult stem cells are scattered across all tissues in the body and are not entirely blank. For example, adult stem cells of bone marrow can form bone and heart muscle cells [114, 115]. Meanwhile, embryonic stem cells are more versatile and can form into any cell type.

The intestines require frequent repairs as the food processing damages the cells that line the intestines. Thus, stem cells always repair the intestines. As mice age, their stem cells do not function and metabolize fatty acids well [116, 117]. However, researchers found that a 24-hour fast improved the functioning of intestinal stem cells in both young and old mice [116, 117]. The intestines of fasting mice healed faster because stem cells improved their functioning during fasts [116, 117]. Stem cells prefer to burn fatty acids as their fuel source [116, 117]. Thus, fasting awakens stem cells and gets them to repair the body as the feasting cycle starts. A fast of 48 hours leads to liver cell regeneration in mice [100]. Researchers need to conduct further studies on whether fasting improves the performance of all stem cells in the body.

Some claim fasting heals the following ailments.

> **Inflammatory Bowel Disease** [9, 35]: Inflammatory bowel disease is a chronic gut inflammation that comes as ulcerative colitis and Crohn's disease. Ulcerative colitis affects the large intestines or colon, while Crohn's disease impacts any tissues between the mouth and anus.

> **Duodenal Ulcers** [35]: Duodenal ulcers, i.e., sores form on the upper part of the small intestines.

> **Intestinal Parasites** [35]: Parasitic worms and one-cell organisms like protozoans live in the digestive system and usually prefer the intestines. The protozoans feed on the gut bacteria, while many intestinal worms prefer sugar as their food. The sources of parasites include contaminated water, undercooked meats, and unwashed fruits and vegetables.

> **Neurogenic Bladder** [35]: People suffer nerve damage to the bladder. They have trouble urinating, urinate frequently, or experience leakage.

> **Acute Glomerulonephritis** [35]: Inflammation damages the kidneys.

> **Pancreatitis** [35]: Inflammation damages the pancreas.

> **Bacterial Infections:** One study showed that mice on an intermittent fasting regime cleared *Salmonella Typhimurium* from their intestines as compared to the non-fasting group [118]. The fasted mice produced Immunoglobulin A, an antibody protein that is part of the body's immune system that clears the bacteria from the intestines [118]. Salmonella causes abdominal cramps, diarrhea, fever, and vomiting. Salmonella poisoning may require hospitalization and antibiotic treatment.

***

I suffered from severe digestion problems that worsened in March 2018. I attended a conference in Bangladesh, and the organizers took good care of me as they fed me five square meals daily. Bangladeshi food is filled with exotic spices and flavors, and the spiciness stings like a mouthful of angry bees. Although the food tasted great, my stomach hurt constantly, and I felt bloated and suffered from constant diarrhea. Since 2017, I gobbled down the Imodium like M&Ms. I took three or more tablets per week, sometimes daily. Also, my weight peaked at 220 pounds (100 kg) with a body mass index of 32%. Thus, I was obese, and, boy, I was in the worst shape in my life.

After returning home, I went on a calorie-restricted diet. On some days, I felt good, and my stomach did not hurt. My stomach hurts a little other day, but it is not like the pain in Bangladesh. Then I started intermittent fasting in April 2018. After six months of fasting, my digestive system's problems disappeared. Now, I take Imodium about one time monthly. Sometimes, I even become constipated, which is a new sensation for me. In the past, every time I ate food, my body always pushed the food out after three hours, sometimes partially digested.

Heart Health

Fasting imparts many health benefits to the heart and blood. For example, fasting reduces blood pressure [9, 11, 14, 17, 31, 37, 50, 51, 106, 119, 120] and slows heartbeats allowing the heart to rest [3, 17, 37, 119]. For example, if fasting reduces a person's heartbeat from 80 to 60 times per minute, the heart gains more rest. (An athlete's heart beats 60 times per minute). Of course, the rest accumulates over time. At 80 beats per minute, a person's heart beats 115,000 times daily. If fasting lowers the heart rate to 60 beats per minute, then that same person's heart beats 86,500 daily – a savings of 28,800 beats. Therefore, the heart can rest and repair damaged structures [3].

Fasting improves blood quality, and the blood feeds the body's heart and other organs, tissues, and cells [3]. For example, medical doctors view low-density lipoprotein (LDL) as the bad cholesterol and high-density lipoprotein (HDL) as the good cholesterol. Since fats and watery substances like blood do not mix, a lipoprotein carries the cholesterol in the blood. LDL transports the cholesterol to the cells, while HDL returns the cholesterol to the liver for disposal [121].

High levels of LDL are associated with a higher risk of cardiovascular disease [11]. Furthermore, medical doctors believe a high ratio of LDL to HDL increases the chance of a cardiac event because the blood has too much bad cholesterol relative to the good cholesterol. Finally, the liver takes the excess glucose in the bloodstream and manufactures triglycerides [11]. Triglyceride is a fat. High triglyceride levels may increase heart disease risk [11]. Then the liver converts high triglycerides into LDL cholesterol [11].

The high LDL cholesterol causes atherosclerosis, which, in turn, leads to heart disease. Atherosclerosis, where cholesterol and fatty deposits build up on the arterial walls, is a problem in our modern society. Children and teenagers show the onset of atherosclerosis at a young age. Atherosclerosis leads to heart attacks when the deposits block an artery that feeds the heart, while blockages of the arteries in the brain cause a stroke. Thus, heart and brain tissues die from the lack of blood and the nutrients that the blood carries.

We start with animal studies to show the power of fasting. In two rodent studies, the doctors deliberately induced heart damage in rats. The rats that fasted every other day had a greater survival rate than the control group [122, 123]. Thus, the stress of fasting strengthens and protects the heart from damage, at least in rats.

The studies on blood chemistry yield different results because of the different genetic lines of rodents that scientists use. LDL cholesterol stays the same or decreases [88, 89], while HDL cholesterol stays or increases [89]. Doctors view the ratio of LDL to HDL as more important. Consequently, the LDL to HDL either stayed the same in fasting mice [88, 89] or decreased [89], which indicates an improvement as HDL becomes larger relative to LDL.

In most rodent studies, the rats and mice either lost or maintained weight from intermittent fasting. However, in two studies, the fasted mice gained more weight than the control group [88, 104]. This study suggests that fasting places stress on the body. Hence, the fasting mice became heavier as their bodies compensated for the stress of fasting. They also ate twice as much food on their feasting day. In addition, fasted rabbits also gained 50% more weight [14].

Numerous studies show patients lose weight and body fat and shave percentage points off their body mass index (BMI) regardless of the fasting regime or whether the people are healthy or obese [31, 51, 84, 106, 119, 120, 124, 125]. However, fasting studies are ambiguous when it comes to cholesterol and triglycerides. Some studies showed LDL cholesterol and blood triglycerides dropping while HDL cholesterol did not change [31, 51, 84, 106, 119, 124, 125]. Some studies showed triglycerides and LDL cholesterol increasing and HDL falling [84, 106]. In addition, men and women exhibit differences in fasting. For example, overweight women witnessed the largest declines in HDL, LDL, and triglycerides during fasting as compared to the control group [126]. Of course, this ambiguity is not troublesome. The reason is simple. The human body breaks down fats and triglycerides during fasting for energy. Then the liver makes ketones and glucose from triglycerides.

Fasting, in theory, reverses atherosclerosis because fasting lessens inflammation while the cholesterol deposits soften [9, 50, 127]. Some believe inflammation triggers atherosclerosis [50, 127-129]. Fasting forces the body into scavenging mode as the body searches for non-vital tissues and materials for fuel. As the deposits and plagues are removed, the greater blood flow nourishes all body organs, tissues, and cells [9, 14]. We are unsure which mechanism clears plagues from the arteries, but some surmise the white blood cells, macrophages, mop up the plaque and utilize autophagy to break down the cholesterol [46, 58]. These white blood cells become foam cells because they look like foam under a microscope. Some researchers believe chronic inflammation causes the foam cells to stick and form deposits on the artery walls [127].

Some claim fasting cures the following heart problems.

> **Angina** [9]: Angina is a severe pain that starts in the chest and spreads to the arms, neck, and shoulders when the heart does not get enough blood. Although not life-threatening, angina serves as a warning for future heart attacks and strokes.

> **Congestive Heart Failure** [35]: Narrowing arteries and high blood pressure weaken the heart. The heart has trouble pumping blood until it becomes too weak and fails.

> ➤ **Thrombophlebitis** [35]: A blood clot inflames a vein and usually occurs in the legs. Thrombus is another name for blood clots, while phlebitis refers to inflammation.

> ➤ **Varicose Ulcers** [35]: Varicose ulcers, i.e., sores usually form on the legs due to poor circulation.

***

I regularly perform a health check once yearly. Every time I have taken a blood test, I consistently scored high cholesterol. Then I always hear the doctor's speech about taking care of myself and the need for statins to reduce my high cholesterol levels. Table 2 shows my cholesterol tests before intermittent fasting. The health measure shows the maximum time a person needs to be healthy. My LDL and total cholesterol were high and exceeded the health measure, while my triglycerides were a little above the threshold.

Table 2. Blood Tests

Measure	Health Measure	Before Fasting	Intermittent Fasting	Intermittent Fasting
Date		2/14/2017	6/7/2018	1/3/2019
LDL	< 100	153	160	178
HDL	> 40	58	49	58
Total Cholesterol	< 200	243	250	265
Triglycerides	< 150	160	207	154
Total / HDL	< 4.5	4.2	5.1	4.6
Blood glucose	< 100	96	89	90

Doctors measure cholesterol, triglycerides, blood glucose, and uric acid in milligrams per deciliter (mg/dL).

I took a health check on 7 June 2018 after intermittent fasting for two months. At that time, I fasted 18 hours twice weekly. I also fasted 18 hours before the medical tests. I wanted to check whether the tests registered any abnormalities from the fast. The urine and blood tests failed to detect abnormalities except that my LDL cholesterol and triglycerides increased while my HDL cholesterol fell. The ratio between total cholesterol and HDL became higher, signaling a cardiac event in my future. The remaining tests were normal.

Dr. Joel Fuhrman observed that fasting patients with atherosclerosis showed a surge in cholesterol levels [9]. Doctors in the Soviet Union also noticed surges in cholesterol at the beginning of a fast [28]. The cholesterol could remain elevated for months because fasting reduces inflammation while the body removes atheromas from the blood vessels. Atheromas are cholesterol deposits in the arteries. Meat eaters usually show a surge in cholesterol, while vegetarians do not [9]. Some claim that vegetarians can fast easily, while heavy meat eaters experience difficulties abstaining from food for extended periods.

I took another blood test after intermittent fasting for 10 months, during which I fasted a minimum of 24 hours twice weekly. I even fasted for 36 hours before taking the urine and blood tests. The urine tests were normal. My HDL increased while triglycerides fell almost to the normal range. Unfortunately, my LDL and total cholesterol worsened. Consequently, I showed mixed improvement.

My doctor did not give me a speech about statins because I showed some improvement in my blood cholesterol tests. Of course, I refuse to take statins because every cell needs cholesterol, as the body uses cholesterol to manufacture hormones and repair cell walls [11, 121]. Furthermore, not only do statins lower a patient's cholesterol, but statins also lower Vitamin D production and co-enzyme Q10. Our bodies produce Vitamin D from cholesterol as the sunlight warms our skin [121]. Meanwhile, co-enzyme Q10, a powerful antioxidant, helps provide energy for our cells and aids in heart health [130].

The 2019 blood and urine tests detected one abnormality – high uric acid. Uric acid is one of the body's most important antioxidants, as it circulates in the blood plasma and scavenges and neutralizes charged oxygen molecules [131]. Uric acid is produced from purines when the body breaks down old cells. In some people, high uric acid causes gout, an inflammatory disease that causes arthritis as crystals form in the joints. Both a high protein diet and fasting raise uric acid in the blood.

I explained to the doctor that I had fasted for 36 hours before taking the blood and urine tests. She looked at me as if I were a raving lunatic. My doctor is Malay, Muslim, and a female doctor, so I informed her I also do 24-hour dry fasts with no liquids nor food for 24-hour stretches. She became even more shocked, as if I had plopped a dead rat onto the center of her desk. By the way, she recommends intermittent fasting with 6-hour eating windows. She thinks fasting beyond 24 hours is too extreme. Good thing she is not a psychiatrist. She would have committed me to the nearest loony bin. Finally, I told her I had written a book about fasting. She wasn't impressed. That is the way it goes. So, I am her crazy American patient.

I also added the blood glucose in Table 2. Although I have not eaten in 36 hours, the body maintains the blood glucose around 100. The following section discusses the importance of blood glucose and insulin.

Insulin and Diabetes

Diabetes, a silent killer, robs a person of their health and eyesight [9, 11] while their bodies feel like a tightly wound yarn ball of aches and pains. Some people with diabetes may lose limbs from amputation and suffer from atherosclerosis, heart disease, kidney failure, and stroke [9, 11, 132].

The hormone associated with diabetes is insulin. We cannot call insulin a culprit because it is not. We possess a flexible fuel system. For our bodies to utilize sugar, i.e., glucose, insulin allows glucose from the blood to enter the cells [11, 12]. The problem with insulin is that the hormone helps the body store glucose as fat.

Some people believe eating copious quantities of sugar is bad for their health. Instead, many people eat various carbohydrates such as bread, pastries, potatoes, and pasta. For the body to utilize the starch in carbohydrates, the digestive system breaks down starches into sugars. Starches are long connected chains of sugar. The ole

Italian saying contains a kernel of truth – to fatten up a skinny kid, feed them large plates of pasta. Some starches, like bread, spike a person's insulin levels more than gulping down pure table sugar [12].

Diabetes, one of the most insidious diseases, originates from utilizing sugar as energy. Diabetes comes in two forms: Type I and Type II. For Type I, a person's immune system mistakenly destroys his or her pancreas, the organ that manufactures insulin [9, 11, 12]. Type I diabetics look skinny and malnourished because their bodies cannot utilize glucose for energy or store glucose as fat. Before insulin injections became widely available, people with Type I diabetes usually died within months after doctors identified their disease.

Conversely, the pancreas functions in people with Type II diabetes and still manufactures insulin [9, 12, 132]. Type II diabetics tend to be overweight or obese [11] and suffer from a range of health problems that doctors refer to collectively as metabolic syndrome, such as insulin resistance, high blood pressure, cardiovascular disease, and diabetes. The diabetic's blood glucose rises to high levels, requiring the person to take additional insulin to lower blood glucose levels. Type 2 diabetics become resistant to insulin while insulin levels remain persistently high [11, 12]. That high insulin level stops the body from utilizing fat as energy.

A diagnosis of diabetes is a sloppy, wet kiss of death. People with diabetes show a gradual deterioration of their health as the disease progresses. At the beginning of the disease, people with diabetes start taking metformin orally, the most widely prescribed medication in the world [9]. As the disease advances, people with diabetes begin injecting insulin directly into their bodies. Over time, people with diabetes require higher and higher insulin doses to reduce their glucose levels [12]. Meanwhile, their health worsens over time, and other health problems appear.

Over time, diabetics' insulin levels remain persistently high, and the cells become insensitive to insulin [12]. Then blood glucose levels rise. People begin putting on weight and become obese, with most of the fat stored around the abdomen. Then people with diabetes suffer from a broad spectrum of problems such as high blood pressure, high cholesterol, and heart disease. Eventually, people with diabetes take half a dozen pills daily to alleviate the multiple symptoms of their disease. Dr. Fung has acknowledged the fallacy in doctor's treatment [11]. The medications treat the symptoms of the disease and rarely cure the patient.

The high blood glucose levels may help fuel the growth of cancers. Both Type I and Type II diabetics experience a higher rate of cancer [133]. As we already learned, cancer loves sugar. Ironically, Type 1 diabetics are more likely to get a cancer diagnosis around the time they learn they have diabetes [133]. Most likely, Type I diabetics learn to control their blood sugar over time, which reduces the incidence of cancer.

In 1915, Dr. Frederick Allen connected the relationship between diabetes and diet [134, 135]. He recommended a high-fat, low-carbohydrate diet to treat Type I diabetes [134, 135]. Dr. Allen also recognized that calorie restriction did not reduce blood sugar levels. Only fasting reduced blood sugar levels in diabetics [135]. He also discovered how sugar and starches contributed to diabetes.

Dr. Frederick Allen treated patients with diabetes at his hospital by following a fast with a calorie-restricted diet [135]. His patients wasted away, which he called inanition. He recommended a shot of brandy or whiskey daily to prevent acidosis. Out of 42 patients, seven patients died. Another study placed a death rate of 78% [135]. We do not know why Dr. Allen did not raise the fat in meals to stop the patients from wasting away during their feasting cycle. Thus, calorie restriction and fasting play poorly with each other because patients will eventually deplete their fat stores and enter starvation as their bodies scramble to find tissues to consume.

Dr. Allen would not survive in today's hostile legal climate, where anyone with money in his or her pockets has a legal bull's eye painted on their back. However, this was the best treatment available until the availability of insulin in 1922. Before 1922, people with Type I diabetes died within months of a prognosis.

We move forward to current times when doctors routinely admonish obese patients to exercise more and follow a calorie-restricted diet to help patients lose weight. The doctors believe that weight loss will correct the person's health problems. As Dr. Fung explained brilliantly, diabetes and insulin resistance originate from a hormonal imbalance and not from weight [11, 12]. If a patient loses a massive amount of weight, the weight loss does not correct the hormonal imbalance. We all know what happens. The weight returns with a vengeance, bringing a few extra pounds for good measure. That way, the dieter is punished for trying to lose weight.

Dr. Fung's observation explains the paradox of the popular TV show *The Biggest Loser*. We all cheered for our favorite contestants as the fierce Jillian and holistic Bob pushed their teams to lose the most weight. The contestants ate healthy, reduced-calorie meals and exercised five hours or more daily. The contestants lost an incredible amount of weight, 100 pounds (or 45.5 kg) or more.

What happened when the contestants returned to their old lives? The weight returned with a vengeance. Exercise and a restricted-calorie diet did not restore the balance of hormones. In one research study, dieters lost weight on calorie restriction [136]. Although their insulin sensitivity improved, their blood glucose levels remained the same [136]. Eventually, they regained their weight after they had quit their diets.

Fasting helps correct hormonal imbalances. Fasting returns glucose to normal levels, reduces the insulin level in the blood, and makes the body's cells more sensitive to insulin [11, 19, 37, 132, 136-138]. Fasting acts like a reset switch. For instance, we must switch off an electrical gadget for several seconds to reset the device. Alas, the body requires a longer reset time. In my case, I need between 24 hours and 36 hours to reset my body's hormones and gain the benefits of fasting. However, each person differs and requires different reset times. In one study, overweight women who fasted became less sensitive to insulin because the body reserves scarce glucose for the brain and nerve cells [126, 139].

One study illustrates the power of fasting to alleviate the symptoms of Type 2 diabetes. The study examined three patients who injected insulin medication for 25 years [140]. They also suffered from high blood pressure and high blood lipids [140]. They fasted three times per week for 24 hours [140]. One patient came off insulin in five days, while the other two took 13 and 18 days to come off their medication [140]. They all lost weight and slimmed down [140].

Intermittent fasting, of course, is a key to long-term weight loss. We fast once or twice a week for the rest of our lives. Hence, intermittent fasting stabilizes our weight. If we stop fasting, then, of course, we will gain weight again. Remember—fasting and feasting are the heads and tails of the coin of life. We practice both to ensure a long, healthy life.

Human Growth Hormone

The pituitary gland, located at the base of the brain, manufactures the human growth hormone (HGH) [141]. HGH helps the body burn fat for energy, build lean muscle mass, and strengthen bone density [11, 17, 141-143]. Other HGH claims include boosting testosterone, hastening healing, and improving sleeping quality [142]. Furthermore, children require HGH to mature into adults. HGH peaks around puberty and continues to decline over a person's life [11].

HGH and insulin are adversaries because when insulin levels rise, HGH levels fall, and vice versa [11, 144]. Furthermore, obese people produce little HGH because some characteristic of obesity inhibits the production of HGH [141]. HGH varies during the day and peaks at night as sleepers approach their waking time [11]. It is also the same time when the sleeper has not eaten anything since their last meal unless they sleepwalk to the fridge for a midnight snack.

Some males inject HGH into their bodies as a fountain of youth. The HGH makes the men look younger and muscular because it builds muscle and reduces fat. Vanity comes with a price. Males pay between $1,000 and $5,000 monthly for HGH injections from a reputable company [142]. Men could take low-cost HGH tablets, but they are less effective than injections [142].

In one study, researchers found that men in their 50s showed strength gains when taking HGH [145]. However, the men's weight and waist size increased after six months [145]. Of course, HGH injections are not as effective as naturally produced HGH. For this study, the researchers used a small sample size. Small samples are a blessing because researchers can collect and measure various biological markers. However, my statistics professor once said that statisticians expand their data sets to find statistical differences. If the experimental and control groups differ in a measure, then a large sample size will likely find a statistical difference. The relationship must be strong in small samples to find variables statistically significant.

We fasters can save our money. Fasting costs zilch. Zero! Nada! Intermittent fasting for least 24 hours boosts HGH production significantly [11, 19, 38, 144]. The HGH is 100% natural, produced within our bodies. The study indicates that we should enter a fasting state before we go to bed because HGH production peaks around 2 AM when sound asleep [144]. We do not need that pesky insulin messing with our vanity.

Psychological Problems

We have already seen the benefits of fasting on the brain, as fasting improves one's mental powers. The fasters' memory, reasoning, and attention span improve [2, 3]. In addition, all senses of the faster become more acute and sensitive. Thus, some fasters feel more spiritual and have a greater connection to religion.

Fasting also treats or alleviates the following psychological symptoms and problems.

➢ **Addictions** such as alcohol, caffeine, cocaine, and nicotine [9, 28]: We should not be surprised since religion warns us of these vices.

➢ **Anxiety** [9, 35]: A person suffers from panic attacks, compulsive behavior, or constantly worries. A related condition called neurocirculatory asthenia causes fatigue, heart palpitations, rapid heartbeat, and shortness of breath. In the old days, we call this an anxiety attack or panic attack.

➢ **Depression** [9, 35]: A person enters a state of pessimism, feels wholly inadequate, or views oneself as a failure. Sometimes, a depressed person thinks about suicide.

➤ **Neurosis** [9, 35]: A person has a mild personality disturbance. Neurosis includes phobias when a person has an intense fear of spiders, heights, or enclosed spaces.

➤ **Psychosomatic Disease** [35]: Some neurotics believe they are sick when, in fact, they are not.

➤ **Schizophrenia** [3, 28, 35]: A person with schizophrenia perceives distortions of reality and thought, and the person withdraws from social relationships.

➤ **Insomnia** [35]: Fasters experience better and more restful sleep.

➤ **Epilepsy and Seizures:** Fasters prone to seizures experience a reduction in frequency or a complete absence of seizures during a fast [3, 14, 18]. Sometimes, seizures return once the faster resumes eating [3].

Some fasters claim enhanced psychic abilities, such as telepathy and clairvoyance [3, 14]. However, no evidence supports this claim. Dr. Herbert Shelton supervised over 30,000 fasts and failed to witness one case of heightened psychic abilities [3]. If intermittent fasting enhanced my psychic abilities, I would have won the lottery at least twice or thrice. Of course, winning the lottery four times or more is too greedy.

Other Health Benefits

The following are some of the ailments and illnesses that fasters claim that fasting has cured. These conditions do not neatly fit into the previous categories, but they are often cited as potential benefits of fasting.

➤ **Rosacea** [35]: Victims suffer from extreme redness around the cheeks and nose [9].

➤ **Chronic Neck and Back Pain** [9, 35]:

> **Osteoarthritis** [35]: The cartilage, the soft cushion between the joints, stops bones from grinding against each other. During osteoarthritis, the cartilage breaks down and allows the bone to rub against another bone. Fasting reduces the symptoms of osteoarthritis.

> **Fibromyalgia** [9, 34, 35]: The sufferers experience muscle aches and stiffness.

> **Gout** [14, 35, 51]: The sufferer experiences a buildup of uric acid in the body that accumulates and inflames the joints.

> **Impotence and Infertility** [3, 14]: After extended fasts, men lose their impotence while women unable to conceive become expectant mothers [3, 14]. Ironically, women experience morning sickness after conception, which forces the women to fast as the morning sickness prepares the body for the pregnancy.

> **Uterine Fibroids** [35]: Non-cancerous growths appear along the muscle tissues of the uterus.

> **Venereal Diseases** such as gonorrhea and syphilis [3, 14].

We do not have a summary of Dr. Shelton's patients to calculate fasting's effectiveness in curing diseases. However, we have the statistics from Dr. James McEachen, who treated 715 patients in a sanatorium near Escondido, California [14]. He treated his patients with fasting between 1952 and 1958, and 294 patients recovered completely or made substantial improvements [14]. Another 360 patients showed modest improvement [14]. Finally, 61 patients showed no improvement [14]. Consequently, fasting healed at least 91.5% of the patients including tuberculosis infections.

In 2019, researchers extensively studied prolonged fasting in healthy people between 4 and 21 days [31]. The study permitted the fasters to consume between 200 and 250 calories daily [31]. From the study, 404 participants reported a health problem, and 84.4% claimed an improvement in their health [31]. Furthermore, only two suffered medical problems during the fast from 1,422 subjects [31]. Thus, prolonged fasting is safe and effective for healthy people and helps improve most fasters' health.

We have read about the amazing health benefits of fasting. Exercise, diet, or medicine does not even come close to imparting the same health benefits as fasting. Fasting smokes all the other alternatives. If we have yet to start fasting, what is stopping us? I am ready to fast some more.

3. Fasting and Longevity

"He who eats until he is sick must fast until he is well."
– English Proverb

In this chapter, we outline the connection between fasting and longevity. Even with our scientific knowledge and technological progress, we do not know why we age. Consequently, we discuss the human lifespan, the current theories of aging, and how fasting influences aging and longevity. Finally, we discuss the Soviet Union because it was the only modern nation to dedicate resources to the study of fasting.

The Human Lifespan

American society has made giant strides in sanitation, refrigeration, and medicine, raising life expectancy. In 1900, men lived on average 46.3 years, and women lived 48.3 years [146]. Life expectancy has dramatically increased, with men born in 2015 living 76.3 years and women living 81.1 years [147]. However, some claim that the American obesity epidemic will erase our progress in longevity as people worldwide become sicker and experience more medical complications.

One problem with aging is that we do not know the life span of humans. However, the Holy Bible provides the answer. Return to Genesis, when God created Adam and Eve as the first humans. God forbid Adam and Eve to eat the forbidden fruit from the Tree of Knowledge. Then God banished Adam and Eve from the Garden of Eden before they could eat the fruit from the Tree of Life and attain everlasting life (Genesis 3 [5]). The Bible clearly states that Adam lived 930 years while his son Seth lived 807 years. Unfortunately, the Bible neglects Eve and her lifespan. The Bible is also vague about whom Seth married since Eve appears to be the only human female.

Once we reach Noah, 10 generations later, Noah's father lived 595 years while Noah lived 950 (Genesis 9 [5]). Here is the thing. God grew tired of man's wickedness and flooded the earth to purge the land of humans. Then God reseeded the earth with Noah's family and set the age of man to 120 years (Genesis 6:3 [5]). Although Noah and his sons lived a long life, the life expectancy began dropping with each new generation after Noah.

We may view the Bible as making a mistake in ages. However, archaeologists found Sumerian clay tablets near the city of Mosel, Iraq. The city is located near the covered ruins of Nineveh, an ancient Assyrian city. The Bible mentions Nineveh several times. One set of clay tablets lists the kings before the Great Flood, with reigns lasting 30,000 years. Interesting huh?

God probably thought humans could not be so destructive to the world if he vastly shortened our lifespans. We showed God. It just took us longer to turn the world into an overflowing, festering trashcan.

We should not be surprised that the 120-year lifespan is accurate. For example, Jeanne Louise Calment (1875-1997), the longest-living person, lived to the ripe old age of 122 years [148]. As a child, she saw the construction of the Eiffel Tower and sold canvases to Vincent Van Gogh in her father's shop [148]. She even smoked cigarettes [148]. She complained about the bland food in the retirement home because she wanted fried and spicy food and ate over a kilogram of chocolate weekly. (So, we have one good reason to eat junk food.) It does not appear she fasted, but life is good with a bit of chocolate, fried, spicy food, and possibly a cigarette.

We are still determining the long-term effects of fasting. Nevertheless, we know the lifespans of four fasters born in the 19th century. They were born at a time with an average lifespan of fewer than 50 years. Mahatma Gandhi (1869-1948) lived for 78 years until he was assassinated. Upton Beall Sinclair, Jr. (1878-1968) and Dr. Herbert Shelton (1895-1985) lived until 90 years old. At last, Dr. Edward Dewey (1837-1904) lived 67 years.

Sinclair wrote over 100 books, mostly fiction, and wrote the famous *Fasting Cure* in 1911. He also wrote several popular newspaper stories on fasting. Ironically, Upton Sinclair did not believe in intermittent fasting [1]. He believed people needed to change their lifestyle and practice prolonged fasts.

Dr. Edward Dewey grew tired of medications and tonics that failed to cure diseases in the 19th century [2]. During his time, medical doctors supplemented medications with whiskey [2]. Dr. Dewey stumbled on intermittent fasting and recommended that his patients skip breakfast daily and eat lunch at 1 PM, which equates to an 18-hour fast [2]. He wrote *The No Breakfast Plan and the Fasting-Cure* in 1900, chronicling patients' stories and how intermittent fasting cured their ailments [2].

Dr. Herbert Shelton started a fasting clinic in Texas. Although he helped cure over 30,000 patients with a variety of medical conditions, one faster died at his school in 1978. The deceased's wife won her negligence lawsuit against Dr. Shelton and bankrupted him [149]. At this time, Dr. Shelton was disabled suffering from Parkinson's disease [149].

The faster who died illustrates the case when a patient is beyond repair. Previous doctors cut out parts of his large intestine and cut into his stomach. The patient wore a sack to collect fecal matter [149]. Even though fasting provides many benefits for the body, fasting has limitations and cannot perform miracles. If a faster needs a miracle, he or she must appeal to a higher power.

The point of this section is that the 120-year lifespan appears accurate although historical texts indicate humans before the Great Flood lived much longer. Unfortunately, scientists and doctors do not know why we age. In theory, we humans should live a long time because our bodies possess remarkable systems to repair damaged cells and tissues.

Theories of Aging

Scientists do not know why we age. They devised many theories to explain it. Many of these theories relate to each other, with the truth lying somewhere in between.

The typical aging theories include the following:

> **The Cellular-Congestion Theory:** The cell accumulates wastes over time, and it is the most popular theory [9, 150-152]. Eventually, the waste overloads and damages the cells [9]. The

wastes come from toxins or free radicals [9]. Of course, a faster switches on autophagy that plays a vital role in cleaning up and repairing cells.

➤ **The Free-Radical Theory:** A free radical, i.e., a charged molecule, damages cell parts. The natural process of breaking down food into energy creates free radicals. They are also referred to as reactive oxygen species, where oxygen becomes negatively charged. Other sources of free radicals come from pollution, toxins, and smoking. People with elevated insulin levels may produce more free radicals that harm the body's cells [153]. Now, we see the importance of antioxidant vitamins because antioxidants neutralize the charged molecules and prevent cell damage [154]. Fasting raises antioxidant substances in the body, like uric acid.

➤ **The Telomere Theory:** Deoxyribonucleic acid (DNA) contains the genetic information to create life or, in other words, the blueprint of life. The cell's nucleus contains DNA. Some cells, like red blood cells, hair, nails, and skin, lack a nucleus with DNA. In addition, DNA resembles two chains coiling together to form a double helix. The ends of the DNA chains are telomeres that tie the DNA together like a cap or aglet at the end of the shoestring. As a cell divides, the telomeres shorten. Like the fraying of a shoestring missing the cap, cells cannot divide once the telomeres become too short. Many cells divide a maximum between 40 and 60 times, called the Hayflick Limit [150-152]. Once aging cells reach the upper limit, they stop dividing and become senescent cells.

The telomere ensures the integrity of the DNA since cell replication causes mistakes in DNA [115, 155-158]. Too many cells with shortened telomeres accumulating in one area could lead to problems with the immune system, organ failure, or cancer [155]. People with metabolic syndrome and diabetes possess shorter telomeres [159, 160].

Cancer and tumor cells become defective and violate the Hayflick Limit [151, 157, 161]. These cells can divide indefinitely, which makes these cells dangerous to the body because cancerous cells produce telomerase, an enzyme that rebuilds the telomeres at the end of the DNA [161]. Scientists believe that by suppressing the telomerase, the cancer cells will reach the end of their life and die by apoptosis, also called programmed cell death [161]. Apoptosis is a cell going through a sequence to kill itself, like the heroes activating the self-destruct mechanism in a starship.

The Telomere Theory is beautiful. For example, women show a slower erosion of their telomere length than men, although both are born with the same telomere length [162, 163]. Women usually outlive men. In addition, people with shorter telomeres and over the age of 60 tend to die sooner from age-related diseases than people with longer telomeres [163].

Lack of exercise, inflammation, obesity, pollution, smoking, stress, and an unhealthy diet could lead to premature telomere shortening [157, 164]. Yes, stress can lead to premature telomere shortening. Thus, we have a connection between a mental state and the health and longevity of a person at the cellular level. Unfortunately, some people are prone to rapid telomere shortening, which causes premature gray hair, cancer, vulnerability to infections, and a shorter life span in adults [157].

As always in science, telomeres fail to account for one critical fact. We expect telomere shortening to cause problems in high-turnover cells in the skin, intestines, and blood. The body always produces and replicates these cells continuously, as living life always damages these cells. Nevertheless, telomere shortening appears in low-turnover cells such as the heart, liver, and brain cells [157, 165]. Something else is purposely shortening the telomeres over time.

> **Senescent Cell Theory:** Cells losing their ability to replicate become senescent because of the Hayflick Limit. DNA damage, or oxidative stress can cause cells to become senescent [44, 115, 156, 166]. The senescent cells produce chemicals that contaminate the nearby healthy cells [156, 158], and some

refer to senescent cells as zombie cells. Hence, a body is a perfectly green lush grass lawn in the spring, and a senescent cell is a sprouted dandelion. By fall, the yard looks like hell with a field of dandelions. This theory explains why a person gets one gray hair; the gray hair grows into a gray patch. The senescent cell tells the neighboring cells to produce gray hair via chemical messengers. The body begins aging as the body accumulates too many senescent cells.

The senescent cells sending off toxic garbage signal the body to kill them via apoptosis. The white blood cells in the immune system gobble and eliminate the zombie cells to remove them from the body. As we age, senescent cells accumulate rapidly, and the immune system becomes overwhelmed and cannot eliminate them [156, 167]. The immune system also becomes inefficient over time. Some believe senescent cells cause chronic inflammation [44, 156, 158, 167, 168] that leads to many diseases that we outlined in Chapter 2.

Scientists discovered one species, the Hydra, that does not experience senescence [169]. We are not referring to the mythical creature with five heads. The Hydra is a simple lifeform living in freshwater. It has an elongated body with tentacles coming off one end. Theoretically, the Hydra does not age as the cells completely regenerate themselves.

> ➢ **Intercellular Communication Theory:** Cells communicate with each other using protein messengers called cytokines. We already discussed senescent cells, which send out chemical messages that turn neighboring cells into senescent zombie cells [156, 158]. Furthermore, a tissue suffering from inflammation sends out inflammatory cytokines that could harm healthy tissues around it [158]. In a Japanese study including 684 centenarians, the researchers checked a variety of factors such as kidney and liver function, glucose and lipid metabolism, and immune cell senescence [32]. They concluded that low levels of inflammation contributed to the long life span [32]. The centenarians also possessed longer telomeres [32].

> **The Cross-Linkage Theory:** As we age, body tissues such as collagen develop cross-links between cells [9]. The tissues lose their elasticity and start functioning abnormally [9]. A body's metabolism creates energy and substances to sustain a cell's life. However, metabolism produces incomplete substances that become wastes in the cell and form cross-links with other cells [9, 115]. Excessive protein intake helps contribute to cross-links [9].

Dr. Joel Fuhrman warned people about consuming high-protein diets, such as those with too many eggs and meat [9]. The body uses protein to build structures, and thus, the protein promotes rapid growth [9]. People and animals that mature quickly also die sooner [9]. For example, children reaching puberty at a younger age will tend to die at a younger age.

> **Genetic-Code-Error Theory:** A cell's DNA becomes damaged from free radicals or cellular congestion [9, 158]. Too many cell divisions cause errors in the DNA. The damage and errors in DNA prevent the cell from splitting itself to create new cells [150, 158]. Even though the cells contain telomerase enzymes to repair the DNA and extend the telomeres, severe damage from free radicals and cellular congestion could prevent repairs [9, 158].

> **Mitochondria Dysfunction:** The mitochondria serve as the cell's energy furnace as they create energy for the cell. As a person ages, his or her mitochondria become less efficient at utilizing energy that slows metabolism and cellular function [158, 170]. Dysfunctional mitochondria leak toxic compounds, free radicals, and reactive oxygen species that damage the components within a cell [41, 115, 154, 156, 158, 165]. In addition, telomere shortening can also lead to poorly functioning mitochondria [165].

> **Stem Cell Theory:** A stem cell is a blank cell. The body can fashion a stem cell into any cell, such as a blood cell or nerve

cell. The body utilizes stem cells to repair damaged cells. As we age, our bodies produce fewer stem cells [115, 158]. Meanwhile, the telomeres also shorten as stem cells divide, which causes the stem cells to function poorly over time [115].

> **Suppression of Autophagy Theory:** We already discussed the importance of autophagy and how the body uses autophagy to rejuvenate and recycle parts within our cells. Autophagy slows aging because the body recycles a poorly functioning cell and makes it healthy again. Thus, the body does not need to kill and replace the cell. Then the body slows the march to the Hayflick Limit by preventing the creation of a new cell as the old cell is revived and restored.

Reduced autophagy leads to accelerated aging in living tissues [41, 158]. Scientists found that as worms, flies, and mice age, their bodies accumulate more Rubicon, a protein [39]. The protein suppresses and inhibits autophagy [39]. Thus, aging causes autophagy to weaken over time [42]. Unfortunately, we do not know if we could increase longevity by boosting autophagy or artificially eliminating the Rubicons.

We have to be careful about age. I was surprised by the fasting results of my landlord in Las Vegas. Bernie is 85, and after talking to me, he started 24-hour fasts twice a week with periodic longer fasts. After two weeks of fasting, Bernie visited his ophthalmologist, who was shocked by Bernie's improvement in his eyes. The doctor asked what he was doing, and Bernie replied that he was fasting. The doctor gave him a blank look as if Bernie rattled off a 19th-century witch's spell for longevity. However, Bernie's second doctor was curious and said she would research fasting. Furthermore, Bernie showed improvements and gains in the gym, and I was looking at him one day. He looked younger. Bernie claims he will live 110, and I think he will make it. The story's moral is that fasting still does wonders at any age. Let us achieve at the 100-year mark or the 120 mark.

Epigenetic Theory of Aging

Deep in every cell in our body is a cellular clock. This clock begins ticking the moment we are born, even though we do not see the effects of time and age until we reach midlife [171], or at least that is the age when aging is on our minds. Scientists call this the Horvath clock, which is named after the discoverer [171].

The cellular clock is associated with our DNA. Our DNA comprises four types of nucleotides, which we can view as building blocks of our life. We view a nucleotide as a molecule that comes as adenine, cytosine, guanine, and thymine [171]. We usually refer to them by the first letter in their name – A, C, G, and T. These building blocks form DNA instructions, equivalent to a computer program. Our cells read the DNA and use this information to build cell structures through transcription.

Our DNA is a digital program similar to computers and laptops. For example, digital computers rely on two states: On or off, or one and zero. These states define CPU functions, such as addition or subtraction, and represent data. Similarly, DNA is composed of four building blocks, giving four states. Again, this is digital information because when a cell reads the DNA, the nucleotide is either there or not. Thus, information is stored digitally in the DNA. Furthermore, we view a gene as a line of programming code to build proteins and structures.

The DNA in every cell has about 6 billion nucleotide pairs. The pairs come from the double helix, which replicates information on two strands that coil around each other. The double helix is essential because when a cell splits into two, the divided cells can rebuild the other side of the DNA with little error.

Here is the thing. We do not want a cell to access the whole DNA program. For example, a skin cell only needs to read the part of the DNA to build proteins and structures that a skin cell needs. The skin cell does not need to build a structure that a liver or heart cell requires. As the cell forms an identity, methyl groups are added to the DNA. A methyl group is a molecule that blocks a cell to read a portion of DNA. That way, a skin cell cannot build a protein or structure that a liver or heart cell would have. These methyl groups give the DNA its identity.

That is where the Horvath clock comes into play. Over time, a skin cell's DNA will add new methyl groups to the DNA, which prevents the skin cell from reading that portion of the DNA. Thus, a skin cell loses the ability to build some needed structures. Then some methyl groups may fall off the DNA. Then that skin cell could read and build a structure for another cell. That is why we have hair growing out of the weirdest places when we age.

A human genome has over 20 million methylation sites, and only a few thousand correlate with age in the Horvath clock [172]. An aging cell loses about 60% of its methylation [172], while a cell can gain an additional 40% in methylation, allowing a cell to build new components [172]. Consequently, aging causes the body's cells to lose their identity through methylation. The Horvath clock measures the addition and loss of these methyl groups. Unfortunately, the story does not end here.

DNA is a long molecule, and the cell wraps it around small protein balls called histones [171]. This process is similar to coiling a garden hose in loops to make the hose compact and ready for storage. However, the DNA is still too long, and the small loops are wrapped around bigger hoops called chromatin, which are wrapped into larger loops known as chromosomes [171]. Consequently, our DNA is wrapped tightly in every cell.

Let us say we are fasting, and the fasting signal is sent to our body's cells. The mTOR switches off while AMPK switches on. These proteins communicate this information to the cell. Each cell has to uncoil that part of the DNA to read what to do when it knows glucose has become scarce. For example, the cells could build autophagosomes and send these little Pac-Men to go around the cell searching for weak structures to gobble and break down into amino acids, which we call autophagy. Thus, fasting activates some genes and silences other genes.

Over our lifetime, methylation causes cells to lose access to some information they need and gain access to new information they do not need. Then all our cells are constantly coiling and uncoiling the DNA to read this information. Eventually, the cell loses the ability to coil and uncoil the DNA to read this information. According to David Sinclair, a Harvard scientist, "Aging, quite simply, is a loss of information [171]." It is a neat little theory, and it explains a lot. Technically, the cells do not lose the information in the DNA. Our cells begin losing the ability to read this information contained in the DNA.

The story does not end here. We have yet to discuss the factor that causes our cells to lose the ability to read the DNA. Researchers have found longevity genes called sirtuins. Most mammal cells produce seven sirtuins that regulate, reproduce, and repair the DNA [42, 171].

The seven sirtuin genes include the following:

> **SIRT1** maintains epigenome control and DNA repair [171, 173]. SIRT1 keeps mice lean, improves glucose tolerance, and lowers blood cholesterol and insulin levels [174-176]. The SIRT1 gene helps lengthen telomeres [171, 175], prevent cell senescence [177, 178], and may delay cell death [168]. Fasting [48, 174, 175] and the ketogenic diet [16] help turn on this gene.

> **SIRT2** controls cell division and healthy egg production [171, 173, 174].

> **SIRT3** is found in mitochondria, which controls energy metabolism [171, 173]. SIRT3 activates enzymes to help mitochondria oxidize fatty acids and produce antioxidants [42, 48, 179]. SIRT3 also may help suppress the formation of cancer [173, 174]. Exercise, calorie restriction, fasting, and the ketogenic diet help activate SIRT3 [16, 179]. Consequently, mitochondria produce more energy, boost metabolism, and increase the human lifespan [42, 179]. Mice with the SIRT3 gene under-expressed have difficulties utilizing fats for energy and have an intolerance to cold exposure [180].

Here is the connection of fasting to our brain health. Neurons require a massive amount of energy, which creates the destructive reactive oxygen species. Those nasty, negatively charged oxygen molecules move around and damage vital structures in the neuron. Consequently, SIRT3 helps our neurons produce energy and keep this energy from damaging the cells. SIRT3 also helps protect against Alzheimer's, Huntington's, and Parkinson's diseases [179].

- ➤ **SIRT4** resides in mitochondria and helps control energy metabolism [171, 173]. SIRT4 may help suppress cancer [174].

- ➤ **SIRT5** resides in mitochondria and helps control energy metabolism [171, 173].

- ➤ **SIRT6** is critical to maintaining epigenome control and DNA repair [181]. SIRT6 can also extend telomeres and package the DNA to protect it from degradation [171, 173, 175, 181]. This sirtuin can also delay cell senescence and extend life [178, 181]. Fasting activates this gene since nutrient deprivation is a gene activator [175, 182, 183]. Overexpressing this gene in animals extends the lifespan [183, 184]. At last, SIRT6 may suppress several cancers [185].

- ➤ **SIRT7** is critical to maintaining epigenome control and DNA repair [171, 173].

The epigenetic theory of aging helps explain why we get old. David Sinclair engineered some mice where he could induce artificial breaks in the mice's DNA. The sirtuins reacted and fixed the breaks. However, too many breaks cause the sirtuins to leave their original spot and not return. Thus, the sirtuins cannot help the cell read the DNA program. Thus, the mice became old prematurely [171]. It is confusing, but it appears sirtuins help loosen the DNA packing so the cells can unravel and read the DNA [171], like unrolling a scroll.

The epigenetic theory explains why some vices, such as cigarettes, are dangerous to the human body. Cigarette smoke produces thousands of harmful chemicals that damage smokers' DNA. The sirtuins go to work to fix this DNA damage. Then the cells age as some sirtuins do not return to their original spot. Thus, smokers look older than they are, and their cells have aged at the cellular level. The constant repairing of their DNA from smoking accelerates aging [171].

The sirtuins require a molecule called nicotinamide adenine dinucleotide, or NAD+ for short [168, 174, 186]. The sirtuins act like a sensor for NAD+ [173, 186]. As we age, our bodies produce fewer NAD+ [186-188]. The loss is not restricted to a few cell types. The lower NAD+ strikes all cells, like the brain, blood, immune, pancreas, and skin cells [171]. Some researchers reported lower NAD+ levels in the neurons for Alzheimer's, Huntington's, and Parkinson's diseases [188].

Aging strikes all cells at the same time through NAD+. The sirtuins make fewer repairs to the DNA; the cells lose the ability to read the DNA, and our metabolism slows. That also explains why, as we age, we lose NAD+ and sirtuin activity and become more afflicted with diseases of aging such as atherosclerosis, cardiac syndromes, heart failure, arrhythmias, high blood pressure, metabolic syndrome, obesity, fatty liver, diabetes, and high cholesterol [176].

Some aging could be reversed. Calorie restriction and fasting can activate the SIRT1, SIRT3, and SIRT6 genes. Furthermore, scientists have found other activators. For example, Dr. Sinclair performed a 2018 study where elderly mice were treated with a NAD booster. The booster activated the SIRT1 enzyme. The elderly mice's blood vessels are pushed into muscle areas with little blood flow [171]. The activated sirtuins improved DNA repair, boosted memory and exercise endurance, and kept the mice lean regardless of what they ate [171].

The sirtuins respond to an energy sensor, the ratio of nicotinamide adenine dinucleotide (NAD+) to nicotinamide adenine dinucleotide (NADH) [48, 168, 189]. (The H in NADH is hydrogen). The NADH loses an electron and becomes positively charged, i.e., NAD+. The free electron helps oxidize glucose and releases its energy in the mitochondria. As glucose becomes scarce in the body, the ratio of NAD+ to NADH rises, and bam, the sirtuins become activated [175, 186]. The NAD+ is critical for sirtuin activity, and old mice with over-expressed SIRT6 genes live longer and healthier [183].

We fasters are always searching for ways to improve our health and extend our longevity. One way is to take precursors to NAD+, which are niacin, niacinamide, and nicotinamide riboside (NR) [168], i.e., forms of Vitamin B3. NR may be the better supplement since the body requires two chemical reactions to convert NR into NAD+, and the cells allow NR to enter easily [187]. Meanwhile, niacin and niacinamide need three steps to make NAD+ [187].

Another popular supplement is nicotinamide mononucleotide (NMN), which is not classified as Vitamin B3. (Please avoid NAD+ supplements because charged molecules are not likely to reach and enter the cells). In one experiment, patients with NAD+ deficiencies showed an 8-fold increase in blood NAD+ from niacin supplementation [190]. Furthermore, mice taking nicotinamide showed decreased skin cancer incidence and lower immune response to ultraviolet rays as their NAD+ levels increased [168].

Other activities raise NAD+ levels, such as calorie restriction, exercise, fasting, heat shocks, and low glucose availability [189]. The exercise type does not matter. Aerobic and resistance training raise NAD+ levels [191]. We should not be surprised since these are the same factors that turn off mTOR and switch on AMPK. For example, the mitochondria need to produce more energy during exercise. Thus, the mitochondria need the NADH to donate electrons, which would raise the NAD+ / NADH ratio [189].

Both fat and glucose burning require NADH / NAD+. However, when cells are submerged in a nutrient-rich environment, they prefer sugar metabolism, i.e., glycolysis. Burning sugar for fuel decreases NAD+, suppressing sirtuins' activity [174]. This observation explains why people suffering from constantly high blood glucose levels are speeding up their epigenetic clocks [171]. Thus, we see why fasting, exercise, and calorie restriction reduce blood glucose and slow the ticking of the epigenetic clocks. There is one issue with the literature. The literature is unclear as to why fat metabolism raises NAD+ levels unless cells do not need as much NAD+ to metabolize fats. The literature also needs to explain why NAD+ levels decline as we age.

Diet is another factor that slows the epigenetic clock. A study showed that nine volunteers eating the Mediterranean diet for one year altered their genetic clocks. The Mediterranean diet centers on plant-based foods, like fruits, legumes, nuts, seeds, and whole grains. (This diet limits the white carbs such as sugar, flour, potatoes, and rice). The participants gained 2.5 years on their Horvath clocks [192]. That is not bad – to age one year and gain 2.5 years. The net gain is 1.5 years. In another study, volunteers participated in an 8-week treatment program emphasizing exercise, sleep, relaxation exercises, and a diet supplemented with phytonutrients and probiotics. The participants gained 3.23 years on their Horvath clocks than the control group [172]. Thus, diet influences cellular aging.

One breakthrough study showed that cell aging could be reversed. Researchers took skin cells and added four genes – Oct3/4, Sox2, c-Myc, and Klf4 [193]. The skin cells reverted to stem cells. These genes are called Yamanaka factors and were named after the researcher Shinya Yamanaka. He was awarded the 2012 Noble Prize in Physiology and Medicine. When these stem cells were implanted into mice embryos, they contributed to their development [193]. In addition, when these stem cells were inserted under the mice's skin, some of the stem cells evolved into tumors and various nonskin tissues [193].

Stem cells are a hit-and-miss. Some YouTube testimonials advocate how stem cells improve their health, while others complain about how stem cells grow into weird things. For example, a woman getting stem cell treatment for facial wrinkles experienced stem cells growing into bone structures in her skin. Remember, cells communicate with each other with chemical and protein messengers. The stem cells may not get the correct message.

Dr. Sinclair and his research team experimented with the Yamanaka factors. They discovered that adding three genes – Oct4, Sox2, and Klf4 caused cells to become younger [171]. That is another breakthrough because they can use a virus to carry the Yamanaka factors into the cells. Then the antibiotic, doxycycline, turns on the genes and causes the cells to revert to a younger age [171]. Two questions arise. How do these genes know which methyl groups to add and remove to reverse the Horvath clock? We also do not know if this treatment method would reverse aging in all cells. What is the point of having a 20-year-old body and a 90-year-old heart? We could look good on the outside, but we wheeze, cough, and walk slowly as that old heart struggles to keep up.

I often wonder if our bodies have a master clock. Every cell has an epigenetic clock built into it. Does that imply we have a master clock that sends a chemical message to all cells in the body? The master clock informs every cell of its age and keeps aging in sync.

The origin of my theory is simple. Researchers observed that as they subjected muscle and liver cells from old mice to a serum made from the cells of young mice, both the muscle and liver cells acted like young cells [194]. The researchers took the experiment further and performed blood transfusions between the equivalent of 20-year- and 80-year mice. The old mice's blood harmed the younger mice because the young mice acted decrepit and old [195]. However, the young mice's blood had little impact on the old mice.

Of course, a company, Ambrosia, offers blood transfusions for older people from the young for $8,000. Perhaps technology has created the rise of modern vampires as the elderly affluent prey on the young and broke.

Non-epigenetic Aging Studies

Although the Epigenetic Theory of Aging explains a lot, several studies have yet to look at the epigenetics of aging because this theory is relatively new. Thus, these studies are in this section. The excellent news is that fasting slows down aging in the following ways.

> ➢ Fasting helps rid the body of wastes and toxins. Fasting forces the body into scavenging mode as it searches for nonvital cells and materials and recycles their proteins and components via autophagy.

> Fasting reduces inflammation [31]. Thus, inflamed cells and tissues stop sending inflammatory messages to nearby healthy cells and tissues.

> Fasting encourages the mitochondria to improve energy efficiency and cellular function [170]. Furthermore, ketones produce fewer free radicals as the mitochondria convert ketones into energy [18, 65]. Researchers observed adverse changes to the mitochondria in healthy men after a 24-hour fast [13].

> Autophagy allows the body to restore and recover poorly functioning cells and thus avoid the creation of new cells. Autophagy slows a cell's steady advancement towards the Hayflick Limit and could limit senescent cells and apoptosis. At last, fasting may strengthen the cells from external stresses and protect the DNA within the cell [37].

> Scientists are vague about the mechanisms that trigger apoptosis and the connection between apoptosis and autophagy. They are not sure if apoptosis and autophagy share some of the identical mechanisms or whether the presence of autophagy stops apoptosis [60]. For some cells, the body prefers to keep senescent cells while quickly killing off other cells via apoptosis [44]. For example, the body does not use apoptosis to kill off cells in the heart and liver. Also, cells using ketones for fuel become protected and less likely to die via apoptosis [18, 65]. Of course, the presence of ketones may provide a starvation message to the cells to switch on autophagy [64, 66]. Consequently, we need more research to understand the role between apoptosis and autophagy.

> Stem cell activity goes into overdrive when a faster resumes eating after a fast [116, 117]. The stem cells divide rapidly and replace the cells lost to fasting [116, 117].

Some patients pay enormous sums of money for stem cell treatment because stem cell therapy repairs tissue or reverses age-related degenerative diseases, such as diabetes, heart disease, Parkinson's disease, and stroke [115], For example, Mel Gibson's father received stem cell treatment in Panama [196] because the procedure is not approved in the United States. The doctors harvest the stem cells from the tissues of the umbilical cord [196]. The father showed improved cognition and eyesight and reduced inflammation [196]. For the treatment to be effective, a patient requires multiple stem cell treatments. However, we fasters need to fast for 24 hours or more, and it does not cost us anything for stem cell treatment.

Researchers have conducted few longevity studies of fasting on humans because we live long. The researchers would need to track humans throughout their lives and record how many times they fasted. A good study would require following people for several years to extrapolate trends. Thus, we must revert to animal studies.

We examine several animal studies with short lifespans on longevity. Although we share similar biological processes with animals, the human body responds differently than animals. The following studies are on mice, rats, and worms since they have relatively short lifespans.

➤ In one study, a 24-hour fast triggered a three-time increase in apoptosis in intestine cells in old rats [197]. Thus, the rat's bodies eliminated the senescent cells or zombie cells. In another study, fasting delayed the aging effects of mice with a genetic defect. The defect caused the mice's bodies to produce higher amounts of senescent cells [198]. Although it appears fasting causes apoptosis, we require human studies to determine whether fasting has the same effect. In addition, rodents have a higher metabolism than humans, so they may be more sensitive to a day of fasting than humans.

➤ Fasted mice lived 33.6% longer than fully-fed mice [199]. Depending on the species, mice starting fasting at a young age live longer, while mice starting at an older age die sooner than non-fasting mice [200]. It is possible in these strains of mice that old mice cannot adapt to the stress of fasting. Furthermore, fasting also helped mice predisposed to autoimmune diseases live longer [199]. In addition, calorie restriction boosts longevity in mice [201], rats, rhesus monkeys, fish, flies, worms, and yeast [202]. Ironically, the fasted mice gained 10% more body weight [199]. Perhaps the mice's bodies adapted to the stress of fasting, or their digestive system became more efficient at processing food for nutrients [14]. Similarly, fasted rabbits also gained weight [14].

➤ Researchers compared a group of rats that fasted every other day to a control group that ate freely. The fasted rats lived longer [203, 204] and weighed less than the control group [108, 203, 204], while both aging and diabetic rats maintained kidney function [205, 206]. Ironically, voluntary exercise had little effect on longevity and weight [108, 203].

➤ Researchers studied the ketone, beta-hydroxybutyrate, on mice's vascular cells that line the arteries [207]. The ketone prevents senescence in vascular cells. Senescent cells cannot replicate, while stress and DNA damage can induce premature senescence [168, 177, 207]. People who practice calorie restriction, ketogenic diet, or fasting produce this ketone as their bodies break fat down. Then the ketone rejuvenates the senescent cells. Consequently, the body can transform those zombie cells back into healthy cells. For this to happen, the cells need to produce telomerase to lengthen telomeres at the end of the DNA strands.

➤ A study showed that intermittent fasting extended the life of worms, i.e., C. elegans, by at least 40% [208]. Yes, we are talking about worms. Nevertheless, the study's importance lies in the researchers identifying the gene, RHEB-1, that regulates a cell's growth and cycle. Animals and humans share the same gene responsible for the mTOR and insulin pathways. The mTOR pathway senses nutrients and serves as the switch for autophagy.

> Researchers found that dietary restriction and intermittent fasting extended the life of worms [209] - the absence of food switches on AMPK that preserves mitochondria [209]. The cells also needed the flexibility to merge or break apart mitochondria to extend life [209]. Healthy cells need fusion and fission for healthy mitochondria. It is like combining (fusion) batteries to get more power and removing (fission) batteries to reduce power. Again, this study is essential because humans also have AMPK, which switches on autophagy.

> Scientists show that as we age, the protein, Rubicon, accumulates in the bodies of worms, flies, and mice and weakens the process of autophagy [39]. By knocking out the Rubicon, the scientists extended the lives of their subjects [39]. In addition, mice on a calorie-restricted diet also showed less buildup of Rubicon as they aged [39]. Logically, fasting should accomplish the identical reductions in Rubicon as calorie restriction since fasting leads to a reduction in total calories.

> Scientists found that as mice age, an inflammatory protein called vascular cell adhesion molecule 1 (VCAM1) accumulates in the blood's plasma [210]. The protein leads to cognitive decline and activity in the brain. By blocking the protein in old mice, the mice acted young again [210].

> Researchers bred mice with a genetic disposition for rapid telomere shortening [165]. Of course, the bred mice exhibited signs of rapid aging while their mitochondria began functioning poorly [165]. The mice also had trouble maintaining stable blood glucose levels during a fast [165]. Thus, the mice experienced trouble while fasting.

At this point, we see why fasting is necessary and how it slows and possibly reverses aging. Fasting rejuvenates and restores damaged cells via autophagy and sirtuin activation and kick-starts the production of stem cells that replace unrepairable, damaged cells. However, no studies linked fasting to a master biological clock. Unfortunately, scientists and doctors have only begun to unravel the human body's mysteries. For example, the decline of NAD+ comes close to a clock, but what causes the body to produce fewer NAD+?

Supplements to Prolong Life

We have already established that fasting imparts many benefits and reduces numerous diseases and health problems. A natural question is whether fasting can prolong a human's life. The 120-year life is programmed into our bodies. Most likely, fasting cannot extend our lives beyond 120 years. However, if Americans live on average to 80, and fasting extends the age to 120. We get a 50% increase in our lifespan, corresponding to the previously mentioned studies of rodents and worms in the last section. That begs whether scientists and researchers can untangle why we age and discover substances that either extend our age or make old bodies young again.

We have this notion that we must drink a special elixir, potion, or medicine or eat a particular fruit to extend life. For example, the Bible mentions the tree of life in the Garden of Eden and how God shortened our lifespan from 900 years to 120. Another example is *The Epic of Gilgamesh*, an old tale about the fifth and most famous king who ruled Uruk in 2,500 BC. Thus, we are talking about a 4,500-year-old story.

The story began with Gilgamesh being 2/3 god and 1/3 human [211]. He went on a quest to search for everlasting life because the gods made him mortal [211]. The 2/3 god is an interesting ratio. In gene splicing, scientists use three parents to overcome genetic flaws and deficiencies when tampering with life.

After several trials and tribulations, Gilgamesh met Utnapishtim, the name of Noah in Akkadian [211]. The Akkadian Empire rose after Sumer. Archeologists believe Sumer was man's first civilization.

Utnapishtim guided Gilgamesh to harvest a plant (or flower) growing under the water with thorns [211]. The plant will make a man young again. With weights tied to his ankles, Gilgamesh plunged into the sea and successfully harvested the plant [211]. As Gilgamesh returned home, he bathed in a well with cool water [211]. Then a serpent attracted to the flower's sweet scent came and ate the flower [211]. It shed its skin and returned to the well [211]. (That damn serpent keeps popping up and causing trouble again. He tricked Eve into eating the forbidden fruit in the Garden of Eden.)

The Epic of Gilgamesh may provide a lesson. Perhaps we are not supposed to become young again. Like Genesis, God kicked Adam and Eve out of the garden before they could eat the fruit from the tree of everlasting life. Thus, we have this inherent desire to search for substances to cure our health and make us live longer.

For example, researchers identified several substances that can extend life, and some of these supplements are inexpensive. The supplements include the following:

➢ **Metformin:** The popular diabetic drug reduces glucose production in the liver, i.e., inhibits gluconeogenesis [101]. It also may reduce the zombie cell's nasty secretions and prolong longevity [167] by activating the SIRT1 protein [171]. The SIRT1 protein activates DNA repair and helps to coil the epigenome around its histone spools. Metformin may also turn on the AMPK pathway that switches on autophagy [42, 58, 65, 109, 201]. One experiment used metformin to regenerate the thymus to improve the body's immune system [212].

I do not recommend that readers take this drug without a doctor's prescription. This drug is cheap. I bought a year's supply of metformin in Malaysia for $30 and took one 500 mg tablet a day. The source of metformin came from the French lilac or Goat's Rue.

➢ **Rapamycin:** What makes this drug interesting is where it was discovered – under one of the giant moai statues on Easter Island. Doctors use this drug to suppress a patient's immune system during transplants. The drug prevents the immune system from attacking the transplanted organ or tissue [139, 167, 171]. Rapamycin also inhibits the mTOR pathway and, thus, switches on autophagy [40, 41, 47, 58, 201]. People are interested in rapamycin because it may reduce cancer, improve health, and extend human life [109, 139]. The drug also helps remove the senescent zombie cells [167]. They refer to these drugs as senolytics, and they are experimental. (Quercetin is an over-the-counter supplement and is also claimed to be a senolytic).

> **Curcumin:** This substance is a polyphenol from the spice turmeric. Although scientists have not identified curcumin as a life extender per se, they study its potential to kill cancer cells [213]. Curcumin switches off mTOR [213], similar to fasting, which would switch on autophagy. Scientists implicate mTOR as another factor that encourages the growth of cancer cells. When constantly eating, we continually activate mTOR, which promotes cell growth.

> **NAD+:** The chemical nicotinamide adenine dinucleotide (NAD+) is crucial in helping the mitochondria produce energy in the cell [214, 215]. As we age, NAD+ levels drop over time [171, 214, 215]. The mitochondria in old mice function like mitochondria in young mice when given NAD+ [171, 214]. The NAD+ supplements boost DNA repair and autophagy (i.e., mitophagy) and prolong life in worms and mice [216]. As we would expect, fasting and the ketogenic diet raise blood ketones and, in turn, encourage the cells to produce more NAD+ [65]. Usually, the cells make NAD+ from vitamin B3, niacin, or nicotinamide. Scientists are searching for NAD+ boosters to extend life and reduce metabolic diseases such as diabetes and obesity [215]. (There are many precursors to NAD+, including tryptophan).

> **Resveratrol:** Many believe resveratrol lengthens and repairs the telomeres on the DNA and turns on the SIRT1 gene, which is involved in longevity [69, 178, 217]. In several research studies, resveratrol enhances autophagy [41, 45, 65, 154] by activating the AMPK [69]. Resveratrol is a polyphenol, i.e., an antioxidant.

Sources include blueberries, cranberries, cocoa, dark chocolate, grapes, peanuts, pistachios, and red wine.

This chapter would not be complete without mentioning my four favorite antiaging supplements:

> **Hyaluronic Acid:** A simple compound helps the body retain water and keeps the skin, eyes, and cells hydrated [218]. It also is a powerful antioxidant [218]. In a Japanese village, the residents eat a purple sweet potato that helps their bodies produce high levels of hyaluronic acid. The villagers often die in their 90s while always looking half their age.

> **Astaxanthin:** Astaxanthin, one of the strongest antioxidants, comes from the alga *Haematococcus pluvialis*. Lobster, shrimp, and salmon get their reddish-orange color from eating this alga. Manufacturers induce stress on the alga to switch on the plant cell's survival mechanism, which creates astaxanthin. Then they crack and extract the astaxanthin. Capelli and Cysewski (2013) wrote a good book on astaxanthin called *The World's Best Kept Health Secret – Natural Astaxanthin* [219].

> **Melatonin:** Sometimes, I have trouble sleeping, especially during a 48-hour fast. I usually take this supplement once or twice a week. I limit my usage so I do not become too dependent on it. Overwhelming a body with a substance may cause the body to stop making it. Although not mentioned in this book, the Circadian rhythm is an important cycle. The pineal gland ramps melatonin around bedtime to help prepare the body for sleep. Melatonin is an antioxidant, prevents apoptosis, and protects neurons [220]. It even helps activate the immune response in tumors [220, 221] but can help grow tumors if taken in the morning, i.e., out of phase with the Circadian clock [220]. Here is the crazy part. It may interact with SIRT1 because SIRT1 affects the Circadian rhythm [220, 221]. Some people take massive doses of melatonin before bed to reap the anti-aging properties.

> **Lingzhi:** The fungus lingzhi grows on dead trees. The fungus has been part of Chinese herbal medicines for two thousand years. The Chinese refer to lingzhi as the "divine plant" and "auspicious plant" because it symbolizes good fortune, happiness, longevity, and wealth. The fungus strengthens the immune system and imparts some anti-cancer properties. The Japanese call it Reishi.

We may want to avoid visiting the nearest Chinese herbal shop to buy lingzhi. Simmering the dried fungus in water for a half hour creates one foul-tasting tea. If drinking a cup of lingzhi daily extended one's life by twenty years, I could not do it. On the other hand, the herbal stores offer a pill supplement made from cracked, fungal spores, which is more palatable. The herbalists claim the fungal spores are much more potent than the fungus. Of course, I loved it whenever I would ask for lingzhi at the herbal store; the Chinese clerk would ask if I had cancer.

We must be careful when shopping and taking supplements. We should be minimalists and try to remove as many things from our lives as possible to simplify them. I stopped taking hyaluronic acid, astaxanthin, and lingzhi because I couldn't feel their effects anymore since I started fasting. Currently, I take fish oil, vitamin B complex (i.e., B3 for NAD+), spirulina, and metformin. I occasionally take melatonin for sleeping problems. I also experiment with exogenous ketones during a fast to strengthen them, and I am experimenting with quercetin.

4. After Effects of Fasting

"The best of all medicines is resting and fasting."

– Benjamin Franklin, Founding Father of the United States

We examined the health benefits of fasting and how fasting not only extends the faster's life but also improves the quality of life. Furthermore, fasting imparts additional effects that last well into the feasting cycle. Finally, we cover the rare side effect that makes fasting dangerous – death.

Allergies and Skin Rashes

Fasting influences allergies. An allergen is an airborne substance such as pollen, dust mites, or mold that forces the body's immune system into overdrive as the immune system neutralizes the substance. Insect bites and particular foods could also trigger an allergic reaction. Consequently, fasting could reduce the following allergies over time.

- ➤ **Allergies** [9, 35]: The immune system becomes super sensitive to harmless substances in the environment. Allergies manifest in a variety of symptoms. The immune system produces histamines to combat the offending substance.

- ➤ **Bronchial Asthma** [14, 20, 35]: The bronchial tubes, where the airway divides into two branches and supplies air to the lungs, become inflamed. A person coughs, wheezes, and experiences shortness of breath and tightness of the chest.

- ➤ **Eczema** [9, 14, 35]: Pollen may trigger eczema, where patches of skin become cracked, inflamed, itchy, and red.

- ➤ **Hay Fever** [14, 35]: A person sneezes and has a runny nose and red, itchy eyes.

> **Hives or Urticaria** [35]: A person experiences an outbreak of swollen, red bumps on the skin.

A faster may also experience bouts of skin rashes. The rashes resemble an allergic reaction, but we are not sure. The body tucks toxins and harmful substances into the fat tissues as a temporary remedy during a person's feasting cycle. During a fast, the body burns this fat and releases the toxins and harmful substances into the body again. Dr. Shelton and Dr. Fuhrman believe skin rashes reflect the body removing toxins through the skin [3, 9].

***

In my case, I am allergic to tree pollen. I suffered from severe allergies in the United States for two weeks when the trees awakened after lying dormant during a cold winter. For some years, the allergies were terrible when I wanted to take a spoon and gouge my eyes out.

My allergies were not severe in Malaysia before 2017. I lived in a tropical country where plant life never goes dormant because Malaysia has two seasons: hot and rainy and hot with little rain. I would experience a mild hay fever every several months when a specific tree started pollinating.

My allergies worsened in 2017 and 2018. Incidentally, I was also sick many times during this period. I chewed the antihistamine tablets like breath mints, taking them at least two or three times per week. Antihistamines worked like a charm, but the main side effect is drowsiness, which no coffee remedy can fix.

I started fasting in April 2018, and my allergies went dormant after eight hours into a fast. My sense of smell sharpened and became more intense. It seemed I wore a garland of tree buds around my neck from the strong smell of tree pollen in the air around me. Unfortunately, my allergies returned within 30 minutes after eating food.

I continued intermittent fasting twice a week. After six months of intermittent fasting, my allergies improved. Subsequently, I was taking antihistamines two or three times monthly. After fasting for four years, I rarely experience any allergies. Once a year, I may have a flare-up. Then I take antihistamines for several days. I also stopped carrying antihistamines.

During my fasting journey, I experienced three bouts of skin rashes. The first outbreak occurred after my first month of intermittent fasting—little, itchy red bumps formed on my arms, legs, chest, and abdomen. The bumps resembled hives. Then a six-inch red rash developed on the left side, spanning across the lower torso and upper abdomen, where my stomach is located. I showed my doctor the rashes, and she was stumped. She took pictures and sent them to a dermatologist. They did not know what it was, but the outbreak cleared after two weeks.

I experienced the second and third outbreaks after the sixth and eighth months of intermittent fasting. The rashes occur when I bust through a weight plateau. The second happened when I lost 26.4 pounds (or 12 kg), and the third at 28.6 pounds (or 13 kg). The second outbreak was a handful of red bumps, while the third was severe, with many red bumps covering my body that resembled chicken pox. However, both incidences cleared after two weeks.

Perhaps Dr. Shelton and Dr. Fuhrman are correct [3, 9]. The body cleanses and detoxifies itself of toxins during a fast. Thus, the skin rashes come from the body ridding itself of the toxins through the skin.

Eating and Satiation

Fasting changes a person's relationship with food. When I fasted for 18 hours twice a week, I could exert control over my appetite during the feasting cycle. When I break a fast, I usually add a treat like a candy bar or ice cream to my regular meal. Since I started fasting, I have eaten more junk food and sweets and drank more sodas. However, I eliminated snacking between meals.

When I started fasting between 24 and 36 hours twice per week, my eating habits veered out of control. I would cycle between periods when I wasn't hungry and times of gorging myself.

We are creatures of habit. I re-established my old eating habits by eating breakfast at 6 AM, lunch around 12, and dinner at 5 PM. I reverted to my old habits to control overeating. Otherwise, I would be caught in vicious cycles of extreme hunger and no hunger when fasting beyond 24 hours. That leads to another tip.

> **Tip #6:** If we experience difficulties eating during the feasting cycle, we shall revert to our everyday eating habits regardless of hunger.

I watched testimonies on YouTube, where bloggers claimed that they ate well after a fast and that the weight melted away from their bodies. I followed their recommendation. I am 54 years old, and sometimes, I eat like a starving teenager, but I continue to shed weight while becoming slimmer.

Hunger makes perfect sense after a fast. Autophagy causes cells to recycle parts within the cell while the body kills senescent zombie cells. Hence, the body scavenges for energy and devours any substance not deemed vital. During the feasting cycle, we must rebuild those lost structures. Similar to a growing teenager, the fasters eat and do not gain an ounce of fat.

Many health gurus and medical doctors recommend that fasters control their eating and eat healthier during their feasting cycle [9-11]. This recommendation is easier said than done. Eating habits depend on the person. Dr. Fung has correctly stated that a hormonal imbalance causes obesity [11, 12]. Thus, we utilize fasting to correct the hormonal imbalance, which corrects our hunger and satiation signals. When the hormones are balanced, the body gives the correct hunger signals for food. Thus, we eat until we are satiated.

I am suspicious of the doctors' and experts' opinions about eating healthier. Is healthy food healthy? Since the dawn of civilization, man used selective breeding to alter the food supply over the centuries. Recently, humans accelerated the process and directly played with the genes in plants and animals through genetic engineering.

Let us take a look at meats. Farmers and herders have bred animals selectively over the centuries. They also altered the diet of animals. For example, cattle eat grains even though their natural diet is grass. Farm-raised fish eat protein pellets instead of algae and small organisms. Unfortunately, the changes in diet alter the composition of meat, such as:

➢ Farmed-raised cattle, animals, and fish are usually fatter than wild animals. The nutrient content also differs. For instance, grass-fed cattle build up five times more omega-3 fatty acids than grain-fed cattle [222]. Omega-3 fatty acids reduce the risk of heart disease. Of course, the nutrients in the meat depend on what the farmer feeds the animals and fish. Unfortunately, a competitive industry causes producers to reduce costs as much as possible by using the cheapest feeds.

➢ Farmers inject cattle and animals with a smorgasbord of antibiotics and growth hormones [222].

➢ Farmers restrict the movement of animals and fish because exercise toughens the meat and makes the meat leaner. Farmers sell meat by the pound (or kilogram), so they lose money if the animals lose weight from exercising.

The animals are, in essence, what they eat. Farmers feed the animals and fish with low-quality feeds, which yields low-quality meat. Then we eat the animals and fish and assimilate what they have eaten. Of course, the farmers choose grains like corn to fatten the animals, which are carbohydrates.

Some doctors recommend that people eat primarily fruits and vegetables and meat sparingly [9]. Unfortunately, farmers have altered the genetics of fruits and vegetables through selective breeding. Farmers breed crops to yield bigger and sweeter fruits by boosting tree harvests. Several examples show how humankind has altered the following fruits and vegetables:

➢ **Carrots:** Carrots were gnarly roots that came as white, yellow, or purple. Today, carrots grow as tapered roots and come as orange and red.

➢ **Strawberries:** Wild strawberries grow to the size of blueberries. Farm-grown strawberries approach the size of apples and oranges.

➢ **Bananas:** We eat sweet Cavendish bananas with soft seeds. The original banana had a starchier texture and was packed with hard seeds. (I tried bananas on Borneo with crunchy seeds. An unusual eating experience.)

Fruits and vegetables contain thousands of chemicals. They pack many nutrients, antioxidants, phytochemicals, vitamins, and minerals. Are all these chemicals safe for the human body? Researchers estimate we eat 1.5 grams of natural pesticides daily, exceeding the synthetic pesticides by 10,000 times [223].

We only hear about synthetic pesticides and not natural ones. We should not be surprised. That is the meaning of life – to grow, create offspring, and die. Plants do not like to be eaten since it prematurely ends their existence. A damaged or stressed plant produces natural pesticides to protect itself [223]. In large quantities, researchers have proven these natural pesticides cause cancer in rodents [223].

Several chemicals that are bad for the human body include:

➢ **Potato:** A potato exposed to sunlight grows a green skin. A chemical, solanine, causes green skin and could make a person ill or sick if he or she eats too many green-skinned potatoes.

➢ **Nightshade Family:** Eggplant, peppers, tomatoes, and white potatoes belong to the nightshade family. Researchers identified 27 natural pesticides in these vegetables [223].

➢ **Cancer Prevention:** Between 1992 and 2000, researchers recruited 521,448 men and women from diverse backgrounds across Europe [224]. The researchers found that eating fruits and vegetables weakly influenced cancer prevention [224].

> **Wheat and Celiac Disease:** We adapted the dwarf-wheat variety in the 1950s for higher yields [12, 225]. Modern wheat contains fewer nutrients than older varieties, and some people are sensitive to the wheat gluten in the dwarf varieties [225]. Their immune system identifies the gluten incorrectly as a foreign invader. Then the immune system attacks the digestive system, causing leaky gut syndrome and chronic inflammation [225]. Some people improve their health just by avoiding gluten.

> **Coffee:** It breaks my heart to write this. Roasted coffee contains chlorogenic acid, neochlorogenic acid, caffeic acid, and caffeine, which are toxins to the body [223].

> **Fiddlehead Fern:** A popular delicacy on the Island of Borneo. The fiddlehead is the curled, new leaf of a fern. The fern contains a toxic, carcinogenic substance.

I tried the fiddlehead fern. It is delicious, similar to French-cut green beans. However, I broke out in severe hives and had severe diarrhea for two days. The diarrhea was so severe that I could not venture too far away from a bathroom. Also, I could not eat anything and drank kefir, similar to yogurt, for two days.

Perhaps fast food is toxic crap to the body and potentially causes health problems down the line, like a poorly running car engine from burning dirty gasoline for years. However, humans have severely manipulated all our food, including fruits and vegetables. Although apples and oranges may be better than a juicy Big Mac, they could cause problems in the body albeit at a much lower level. How do I know? All foods elicit an insulin response except pure fats [12]. Of course, nobody eats pure fat. However, both carbohydrates and proteins spike insulin levels [12]. Although not replicated here, dieters can refer to the insulin index that measures a body's insulin response to food. The insulin index is similar to the glycemic index, which measures a person's response to glucose.

The results of the insulin index are shocking. The researchers compute an insulin score for subjects eating 250 calories of a specific food [226] and measure the insulin response over two hours

[226]. For example, white bread scores 100 on the insulin index, while yogurt, which many consider healthy, scores 115 [226]. Baked beans come in at 120 [226]. Fruits such as apples, bananas, oranges, and grapes range between 59 and 82 [226]. Finally, eggs and cheese score 31 and 45, respectively [226].

For another example, many report the health benefits of a juice fast, but the juice fast is weaker than a water fast. Thus, the digestive system breaks down food, which inflicts problems on the body. However, we need the nutrients and energy to sustain life even though fruits and vegetables contain natural pesticides and may not prevent cancer.

Do not get me wrong; we should eat fruits and vegetables for plenty of vitamins and minerals. However, eating fast food occasionally is not the end of life. For example, a health guru, Blake Horton, demonstrates the power of fasting and shows his extreme eating on YouTube, where he eats his mountain of food from a large platter with a layer of French fries covered with melted cheese and small pools of glistening oil. His meals contain between 4,000 and 5,000 calories. Although he cooks his meals and controls every ingredient, he demonstrates the power of fasting. His eating window spans one hour while he fasts for the other 23 hours in the day. He is in shape and athletic-looking, although he shocks viewers with his eating regimen.

That's why I do not worry about indulging in sweets and junk food occasionally. I gravitated towards the Keto desserts, which I find delicious. However, we can transform our indulgence into a reward. If our weakness is a slice of chocolate cake with a scoop of ice cream, a candy bar, or a cream-filled doughnut, we reward ourselves for fasting. Then we sit down and savor that weakness as we break a fast. The taste buds are sensitive to taking 16 hours or more of pause from food; that first bite is a taste of heaven.

> ➢ **Tip #7:** Diets do not work because they punish the dieter. We make fasting work by turning a food weakness into a reward. When we fast for 16 hours or more, we deserve a treat. A candy bar, ice cream, or a can of soda tastes fantastic after a fast. (Keto desserts would be better). That way, we have something

to look forward to when we begin our feasting cycle. Please note that the indulgence is not a tub of ice cream, a box of doughnuts, or liters of soda. We revert to our old eating habits and toss in a treat as a reward.

Because of fasting, I recovered my teenage metabolism when I could eat anything and not gain weight. I violate all the rules that the medical profession advises against. Although I am a rebel by nature, I save the bacon grease. I eat one or two fried eggs cooked in bacon grease daily. I drink the salty brine leftover from my Ramen noodles to ensure I get plenty of salt. I drink cream milk for breakfast. I love fried chicken skin, which is the best part of the chicken. Finally, I sometimes say yes to the whipped cream on my Starbucks Frappuccino.

I have been fasting for over four years, and it has become second nature. Most times, I feel no difference between a fast and a feast. However, I sometimes end fasts with a Big Mac and fries or a bag of Doritos with a Snickers. I revert to my regular eating patterns for my second meal after breaking a fast. Do not worry; I have an atrocious diet, but I fast and exercise, so two out of three is not bad.

I am gradually improving. I do eat some healthy food, and I give the readers some of my favorite salad recipes in Chapter 9. I also eat more fruits, such as blueberries, cherries, strawberries, oranges, dragon fruit, and rambutans, and I made my New Year's Eve resolution to eat healthier in 2022. However, all food contains toxins and natural and synthetic pesticides that could harm our health. The best advice is to eat various foods, especially nutrient-dense foods packed with vitamins and minerals.

Metabolism and Weight Loss

A person usually loses about a pound (or 0.45 kg) of fat for a full day of fasting [3, 9, 14]. The weight loss can drop to ½ pound (or 0.23 kg) daily [3, 9]. However, weight loss varies with the person. Both obese and athletic people lose more than a pound (or 0.45 kg) daily [3]. For example, fasting obese people can lose between 1.5 and 5 pounds daily [21]. In one study, fasters lost up to 9% of their body weight, with significant decreases in body fat within five months [23]. Dr. Shelton claimed that losing much weight during a fast indicates a sick body, while little weight loss means a healthy body [1, 3]. We covered the health benefits of fasting in Chapter 2.

A faster could lose more than a pound daily as the body rids itself of excess water during a fast [3, 9, 11, 17]. When we burn glycogen, our bodies release water [13]. In addition, the lower insulin levels allow the body to rid itself of excess salt and water via urination [11, 17, 227]. When we step on the scales, we smile because we think we have lost much weight. However, we will regain the water weight once we start our feasting cycle again. That leads to another good tip.

> **Tip #8:** We weigh ourselves towards the end of a fast. That way, we do not feel depressed if we have gained several pounds (or kilograms) from water weight. We should also use the scale to determine when we will end the fast. Please note that we could gain weight during a fast by drinking too much fluids. The one measure that never lies is the tightness of a belt.

We do not know at this time whether an obese person losing massive amounts of weight rapidly from fasting will suffer from excess skin. For obese people, losing weight is a double whammy. An obese person loses tons of weight but then suffers from the skin that drapes from his or her body like curtains. Usually, loose skin comes from a 50-pound (or 22.7 kg) or more weight loss. In theory, fasting should cause the body to recycle the excess skin, but more research is needed.

Intermittent fasting boosts metabolism and burns more energy, allowing fasters to lose weight. Fasting boosts metabolism in the following ways:

> Fasting increases adrenaline, i.e., the neurotransmitter norepinephrine that stimulates metabolism [11, 12, 23]. A neurotransmitter is a chemical that allows a brain neuron to communicate with another neuron. Adrenaline is part of the fight versus flight response as it constricts blood vessels and

raises the heartbeat. Consequently, adrenaline prepares the person for action, i.e., search for food because the body's cells are hungry.

➢ Fasting causes the liver to produce glucose from amino acids, called gluconeogenesis. The chemical conversion requires energy, which boosts a faster's metabolism [23].

➢ Fasting boosts human growth hormone (HGH), lowers blood insulin, and helps the body burn fat for energy [10, 11]. Fasting boosts metabolism by 3% [10, 11].

➢ The metabolism revs up after the faster resumes eating. The body must rebuild the tissues and cells lost during the fast from autophagy and apoptosis, the death of old cells. The stem cells go into overdrive to replace the dead cells.

Another reason for the boost in metabolism is that the body has access to the fat stores during fasting. For example, I weighed 220 pounds (or 100 kg) at the worst time in my life in 2018. My body mass index (BMI) peaked at 32.7. That means I was obese with my body comprising about 32.7% of fat. I walked around with 71.9 pounds (or 32.7 kg) of fat with enough fat stores to last at least 71 days. How could my body be hungry for energy, as fasting makes 71 days of energy available?

A person's metabolism relates to his or her mitochondria, the energy furnaces of the cells. One theory of aging suggests that mitochondria become inefficient at utilizing energy over time, which is why we feel colder and eat less as we age. (Remember we discussed SIRT3, which is involved with energy metabolism). Fasting improves the functioning of mitochondria and revs up the energy consumption within the cells [18].

A person consuming a carbohydrate-rich diet overloads their system with sugar because the digestive system breaks carbohydrates like starch into glucose. Consequently, the mitochondria become accustomed to burning glucose for fuel instead of fat. If we always snack every two hours, especially carbohydrates, our mitochondria are stuck burning glucose for fuel.

Fasting switches a person's body from a sugar burner to a fat burner. A sugar burner only lasts two hours before they need another snack or sweet drink. Meanwhile, a fat burner can go hours until the next meal. Thus, fasting makes the mitochondria more flexible in fuel sources as fasters switch back and forth between fasting and feasting.

We see the problem of modern-day society. Doctors advocate eating or snacking every two hours while awake. Some people even wake up during the night and snack. Hence, most people rarely enter the fasting state, or if they do, they awaken and eat to re-kick the feasting cycle again. Thus, the pancreas always produces insulin, so the body's cells turn the glucose into energy and fat. Then people trap themselves in fat storage mode and encourage their mitochondria to burn glucose for fuel. Thus, modern society causes people to be stuck in sugar-burning mode. That also explains why when I tell a person that I fast or talk about ketosis, I get the crazy eye look. If a person never enters ketosis, how else can they burn fat?

***

I tried Adkin's Diet and calorie restriction several times. I have always been good about working out in the gym. I jog two or three times per week on the elliptical trainer and do resistance training twice per week. I jokingly call it my natural health insurance. Of course, my health insurance is much better than the health insurance plan that President Obama and Congress pushed onto Americans in 2010.

I did not know it then, but I ate nothing between 6 PM and 6 AM the next day when trying to get into shape. Thus, I fasted 12 hours daily. My largest weight loss was 11 pounds (or 5 kg). That's it. That was in 2016. Then I became fatter in 2017 as I regained all my weight plus a couple of extra pounds as punishment for trying to lose weight. In 2017, I could not lose weight on calorie restriction, while my weight remained at 220 pounds (or 100 kg).

I rarely dieted because I knew one critical fact—dieters lose weight in the beginning and then regain the weight plus several extra pounds for good measure. I tried calorie restriction and frequent small meals. The calorie restriction left me hungry all the time. I also tried eating small meals every two or three hours, a trick bodybuilders use to build muscle and shed fat. That failed, too. The frequent small meals keep the body in sugar-burning mode.

Then I saw the videos on YouTube comparing calorie restriction and fasting. Later, I learned how fasting switches on autophagy. Thus, I gave fasting a try. At first, I tried 18-hour fasts once per week. The first several times, I thought I would die. I became dizzy when I stood up, and I suffered hunger pangs. Each time I fasted, the process became easier and easier. Then I expanded fasting to twice per week and gradually increased the duration.

The weight loss is miraculous, and I still eat three square meals daily during my feasting cycle while expanding my portion size. I lost 11 pounds (or 5 kg) within a month. The following month, I lost another 4.4 pounds (or 2 kg). Then fasting became interesting. I modified my exercise regime to include fasting. I jog twice weekly, do resistance training twice weekly, and fast twice weekly with one day of rest.

The weight loss slowed each month as I kept hitting weight plateaus. After 7 months of fasting, I lost 28.6 pounds (or 13 kg) with little effort. I weigh 191.4 pounds (or 87 kg), while my waist shrank from 38 to 33 inches. Wow! I wore a 33 in high school and never dreamed I would wear 33 again. My body mass index (BMI) dropped from 32.7 (obese) to 28.4 (overweight). That blew my mind away. Hence, I had to write a book about it. Of course, I am more than happy to be overweight than obese by the government's standards, but damn, I can fit into 33-inch jeans again.

Of course, I almost returned to my college weight of 185 pounds (or 84 kg), the lean years, not the chubby years. Like the other freshmen, I gained the freshman 10 during my first year in college. (The 10 stands for 10 pounds (or 4.5 kg) of weight gain.) That was during the 1990s; now, they call it the freshman 15. The university cafeterias feed the students like cattle ranchers fattening the calves at mealtime.

I have no desire to do extended fasts. I incorporated a lifestyle change, and I plan to maintain my weight loss. Thus, I maintain two fasts ranging between 24 and 48 hours during the week unless I gain a pound or two from my atrocious eating habits. Then I may add an extra fast during the week to correct my weight. I also add at least two bouts of dry fasting to my monthly fasting regime to maximize my health benefits.

That is what blows the mind about fasting. We go through life and put on a little weight with an expanding waist size. A gradual weight gain is part of the aging process. The aches and pains start to accumulate, and our health gradually declines. We know now that we do not have to age like this. We can use the power of intermittent fasting to improve our health and maintain a healthy weight as we age gracefully.

An Accidental Athlete

Fasting enhances the functioning of cells, tissues, and organs. It causes the body to become better adapted to build muscles and recover quickly from workouts [38]. Consequently, fasting improves athletic performance as it transforms anyone into an athlete. Then we use our bodies to play and participate in sports. Thus, all fasters should work out. Fasters should add resistance training to combat muscle loss during fasts [125] and exercise aerobically to strengthen cardiovascular systems.

Once we adjust to intermittent fasting, we can exercise while fasting. Upton Sinclair, the American writer, walked four miles every morning and worked out in the gymnasium while fasting [1]. He also hiked and rode his horse more often [1]. During the outdoor walks and hikes, he exposed his skin to the sunlight, which allowed his body to produce vitamin D while breathing the fresh country air.

I never considered myself an athlete, even though I jogged and lifted weights in the gym since college. I figure that exercise is my personal healthcare plan. Then I began intermittent fasting and witnessed its shocking side effects.

I, for example, have been running on an elliptical trainer in the gym since 2017 because jogging causes too much pain in my legs. I weighed 220 pounds (or 100 kg), and my heavy weight was flattening and crushing my feet. Then I ran on the elliptical trainer for 45 minutes three times per week. Unfortunately, my gut would jiggle as I ran on the machine. Sometimes, after the run, I was wiped out. I would return home and lights out as my head hit the pillow.

I expanded my exercise routines to include charity runs and participated at least six times yearly, ranging between 1.9 and 7.5 miles (or 3 km and 12 km). I had nothing but trouble with the 10 km. I needed to take a break and walk for 10 minutes several times to cross the finish line. The 12 km was worse. I had only 2 km to go, but I could not run anymore. I had to crawl to the finish line. After the races, I felt terrible. Every muscle in my body hurt; muscles that I did not even know I had hurt as if I smashed them with a sledgehammer. Then I suffered for days in pain and agony as I gobbled down the aspirin.

Then I started intermittent fasting twice per week. I run only twice per week; sometimes, I run during a fast. The 45 minutes on the elliptical trainer is nothing. My gut stopped jiggling. After showering, I feel like I did not even work out. In 2018, I ran my first 10k run with no walking breaks. Meanwhile, I walked once for ten minutes in the 7.5-mile (or 12 k) run but completed the race with a good time. I also recovered much quicker after the race, with a fraction of the pain. Now, I skip the aspirin for minor aches and pains.

I had a long way to go before running the marathon, but my students gave me some sour looks as I passed them at one charity run at the university. They never expected uncle, who is twice their age, to smoke them during a race. The Asians reserve uncle to describe older men, while auntie stands for older women. I like the term uncle much better than grandpa.

Fasting improves athletic performance in other areas. For example, I also lift weights in the gym twice per week. Since I started fasting, I lift more weight with more repetitions. Moreover, I am more focused and have better control over my buoyancy when scuba diving. Buoyancy is one of the essential skills in scuba diving. The diver adjusts the air in the BCD to allow him or her to hover above the coral. Improper buoyancy means the diver would bump and scrape against the coral, possibly damaging life forms or floating to the surface too quickly, causing nitrogen to bubble in the scuba diver's blood.

Becoming Younger

Autophagy recycles cell parts, while autolysis removes unwanted tissues and cells. Fasting eliminates the senescent, i.e., zombie cells, and recycles the components. Intermittent fasting once or twice weekly is like working on a classic car. Fix a part here and replace another part there. And bam! Six months later, we drive around the town in a completely restored 1969 Ford Mustang. As we drive by, the engine roars while the exhaust rumbles. Hence, we become young again.

It is not just a modern trend. The effects of fasting on physical appearance have been observed for centuries. For instance, people have long claimed that Mahatma Gandhi looked 25 years younger after a fast [3, 14]. This is because fasting rejuvenates the skin and improves skin blood circulation [3]. Blemishes, blotches, and pimples also clear [3, 14], while wrinkles and fine lines smooth and disappear [3, 14]. So, it is not surprising that fasting can make us look good, young, and sexy.

I am shocked by the transformation. People tell me I look 15 years younger. However, the reader can be the judge. Figure 1 presents three pictures of when I was 40, 50, and 51. The middle picture represents the worst health of my life. The third picture shows the impact of 10 months of intermittent fasting.

I was shocked by looking younger and I also had a dozen red bumps scattered across my body. All the bumps have disappeared. I even had one bump on the back of my right leg for 15 years. One day, I used a band-aid to press a cotton ball saturated with iodine against the abscess to burn it off. It burned for several hours, but the abscess reappeared after the scar had healed. After six months of intermittent fasting, all the bumps and abscesses are gone – dissolved and recycled. Good riddance!

One aspect of aging is that the senses become dull. However, fasting improves eyesight and hearing [2, 3, 9]. I cannot vouch for hearing. Although I have been turning the volume down on my Walkman while listening to classic rock music, it is a far cry from being scientific. However, I worry about the deterioration of my eyesight, which I have kept track of.

Figure 1. My Pictures at 40,50, and 51.

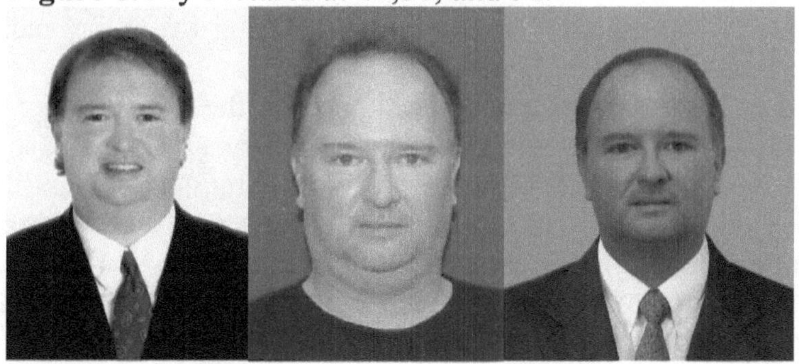

I am farsighted, which means I can see objects far away but not close. Therefore, I wear glasses when I read and, of course, I wear thick, Coke-bottle glasses. At least if I get lost in the forest, I can always use my glasses to start a campfire. The thick lenses would concentrate the sunlight into a laser beam to start a fire.

I provide four eyesight measurements in Table 3. The first was when I was a young man. The second measurement shows my worsening eyesight in 2017. The third shows my vision after 10 months of intermittent fasting, while the fourth is my vision in 2022.

Table 3. Eyesight Measurement

Date	31 March 1995	15 April 2017	8 January 2019	20 January 2022
	Spherical Power	Spherical Power	Spherical Power	Spherical Power
Right eye	+3.00	+4.75	+4.25	+3.25
Left eye	+3.25	+5.50	+5.25	+3.50
	Cylinder	Cylinder	Cylinder	Cylinder
Right eye	-1.25	-1.25	-0.50	-0.25
Left eye	-1.25	-1.25	-1.25	-0.25

Spherical power is the lens power to restore my eyesight to 20/20 vision. The plus means farsighted, while the negative means nearsighted. As we can see, I had terrible eyesight in 1995, with a spherical power of 3 and 3.25. By age 49, my left eye's vision had deteriorated significantly. Since my eyesight is quite bad, the lenses do not correct my eyesight to 20/20 vision. Otherwise, they would be too thick. Consequently, intermittent fasting has improved my vision since the spherical power has fallen.

I also have astigmatism, which means the eyeballs are not perfectly spherical. Astigmatism causes blurry vision because the lens focuses the light improperly on the retina. The cylinder measures the degree of astigmatism. Thus, as Table 3 shows, intermittent fasting has reduced the astigmatism in both eyes. In 2022, the optometrist surprised me during my last visit because I no longer needed bifocals and custom-made lenses. The astigmatism has been corrected enough that I can use standard lenses off the shelf: no more bifocals and expensive lenses.

The last aspect of aging is gray hair. I had little gray patches around the sideburn, a salt and pepper beard, and white hair on the upper chest. After intermittent fasting, I noticed fewer gray hairs, especially on my beard. Thus, fasting is reversing that aging clock by a little.

Senescent cells could be responsible for gray hair. A senescent cell means it cannot divide as it has reached the end of its life. Unfortunately, the senescent cell does not die quietly. It must create proteins and garbage that contaminate the nearby healthy cells, like an elderly person creating a ruckus at the nursing home. That is why we notice a gray strand here and there. Then several months later, the single gray hair grows into a patch of grayness. Hence, fasting helps us look young by triggering the death of senescent cells, which scientists call apoptosis.

Fasting, unfortunately, has little impact on baldness. A person can quickly lose 100 strands of hair daily, and fasting slows hair loss [3]. Nevertheless, I do not know whether fasting has slowed my hair loss, but my baldness has not reversed. I could be sad about the hair loss, but I consider myself lucky since I started going bald in my late

40s. Unfortunately, baldness strikes some men in their 20s as life takes jabs at young men's virility at the prime of their lives.

Fasting has a powerful effect on the body but little impact on dihydrotestosterone (DHT), the hormone responsible for baldness. Scientists believe DHT causes the hair follicles to shrink on a man's head, which chokes the growing hair [228]. Over time, a man's hair recedes in the front, while a bald spot grows on the top of the head. Scientists believe men inherited baldness through their genes [228]. Lastly, balding men are more susceptible to an enlarged prostate, diabetes, heart disease, high blood pressure, and obesity [228].

Drug Testing

Fasting may have one negative side effect. We fast and improve our lives, but the next thing we know, our history comes back to haunt us. What are we referring to? Drug testing.

Fasting allows the body to consume the fat and remove toxins and wastes from the cells. A faster with a previous history of drug use can release those toxins and wastes into the body again. Table 4 shows the testing windows for standard drugs. One pattern emerges: the body metabolizes and expels most drugs relatively quickly within a week for the urine test, with alcohol being eliminated the quickest. However, the body can take up to a month to remove the metabolites of marijuana. As we can see, the urine drug test is biased towards marijuana use.

The problem with marijuana is that the fatty tissues absorb the metabolites of marijuana [229]. Consequently, the more the user smokes, the more substances and chemicals of marijuana get stored in the fat tissues, like charging a battery. Then there is a story of an obese, heavy user of marijuana testing positive up to six months after going clean.

Unfortunately, we cannot control when we take the tests. As Table 4 shows, some drugs have short testing windows, so employers have an incentive to conduct random drug tests unless we are new employees. Although I live in Malaysia, a new employer required me to take my very first urine drug test in March 2019. (It's no big deal—I do not use drugs.)

Table 4. Drug Testing Windows

Substance	Urine Test	Hair Test
Alcohol	10 – 12 hours	NA
Amphetamines	2 – 4 days	Up to 90 days
Methamphetamine	2 – 5 days	Up to 90 days
Barbiturates	Up to 7 days	Up to 90 days
Cocaine	1 to 8 days	Up to 90 days
Marijuana	1 to 30 days	Up to 90 days
Opiates – morphine	2 to 5 days	Up to 90 days
Opiates – Heroin	2 to 3 days	Up to 90 days

Source: Hadland, SE and Levy, S. 2016. Objective Testing: Urine and Other Drug Tests. *Child and Adolescent Psychiatric Clinics* [229]

The urine tests are relatively cheap and the most common [229]. On the other hand, hair tests have testing windows up to 90 days, depending on the length of the hair specimen [229]. Even though employers would prefer the longer testing windows of the hair test, the test may not detect new or infrequent drug use. In addition, blood drug tests are not so usual. They arise during medical treatments and surgeries or when a person is arrested and facing criminal charges. The blood test can determine which drug the person took and the dosage. Finally, saliva tests are becoming popular. For example, we are walking through immigration in a foreign country, and the next thing we know, an immigration officer sticks a cotton swab in our mouth and takes a generous specimen of spit. Fortunately, saliva drug tests have short windows of up to 48 hours for all drugs [229], while marijuana's test window is only 24 hours [229].

The moral of the story is that we do not use drugs. If we have used drugs in the past, we use fasting to clean and detox our bodies and fashion ourselves into better people. However, a faster with a previous history of heavy marijuana use has every right to feel nervous about an impending urine drug test.

Extreme Fasting and Enlightenment

Followers of Christianity and Islam use fasting as a means to commune with God. On the other hand, Buddhists utilize fasting to achieve enlightenment and higher levels of consciousness. Buddhism was founded by Gautama Buddha, who renounced his life as a prince and sought the path to enlightenment. He studied various altered states of consciousness, such as meditation, sensory deprivation, mind control, breathing techniques, and extreme fasting. When he fasted, he ate a cup of vegetable soup with 25 calories daily [230]. Unfortunately, he pushed fasting into starvation with massive losses of body fat and muscles [230]. He also suffered from diarrhea, hair loss, stomach atrophy, and vitamin deficiencies [230].

Gautama broke his fast on the verge of death and experienced enlightenment [230]. A pedestrian offered Gautama a bowl of rice pudding made from milk, rice, and sugar, which broke his fast [230]. After consuming the meal, Gautama entered an intense spiritual state that lasted nine hours [230]. He lived past lives, experienced rebirths in various forms with different moral traits, and passed through heaven and hell [230].

Researchers believe extreme fasting altered Gautama's brain chemistry. As he ate the rice pudding, a meal rich in carbohydrates and milk, the carbs and tryptophan from the milk overstimulated the serotonin in his brain [230]. Serotonin has a powerful effect on mental states. For example, a deficiency of tryptophan reduces serotonin in the brain leading to anxiety, depression, and poor cognition in patients. On the other hand, overstimulation of serotonin leads to hallucinations. The psychedelic drug, lysergic acid diethylamide (LSD), overstimulates serotonin, leading to hallucinations and vivid sensory experiences. Consequently, extreme fasting combined with refeeding caused Gautama Buddha to experience higher levels of consciousness and spiritual enlightenment or gave him one hell of a natural psychedelic trip.

Another form of extreme fasting comes from Lord Mahavira, the "Great Hero," who founded the Jain religion roughly the same time as Buddhism in the 4th century BC in northern India [7]. The Jain religion shares many similarities with Buddhism. The followers deny themselves of earthly pleasures to achieve spiritual purification and enlightenment [7]. The Jain monks and nuns spend most of their time praying, confessing, meditating, and engaging in other rituals [7]. They also fast regularly [7].

The Jain followers respect all living forms and will do their best to avoid harming or injuring any life forms, including insects [7]. They view harm or injury to a living thing as a form of violence [7], which is why they inspect their clothing periodically to remove insects [7]. They are also vegetarians because meat comes from the killing and slaughter of animals.

The followers believe a vegetarian diet is healthier than an omnivorous diet [7]. They avoid stimulating and flavorful food because delicious food is addictive, dissipates energy, and dulls the senses [7]. In addition, a restricted diet helps the Jains clean, purify, and strengthen their body and help purify the soul [7]. They also slim down while their body becomes harder and stronger [7]. At last, they are less prone to sickness, require less sleep, have weaker sexual urges, and have less desire for food [7].

As the Jains fast, they believe their desires and volitions wither away [7]. Consequently, the fast helps the followers remove karma from the soul [7] because karma reflects cause and effect. When we do bad things in this life, these bad acts follow us into the next life. Of course, we can choose to do good deeds and actions that lead to better karma in the future. From the Jains' perspective, removing karma allows the soul to become free and omniscient [7].

Here is where fasting becomes extreme. The Jains believe they will attain enlightenment if they die during meditation [7]. They call this practice samadhi-maran – death while meditating [7]. The follower sits and meditates quietly as he or she waits for death [7]. For example, Amarcand-ji was an old man who fasted until his death [7]. He fasted for 36 days for his last fast, with the last 24 days being a dry fast [7]. Amarcand-ji was talking, sitting, and praying on his last day. Then he blurted, "Now, I will die. [7]"

At his death, people claimed there was a rain of saffron, while his skull cracked open as a wound appeared on his head [7]. Usually, a son cracks his deceased father's head to liberate the soul from the body [7]. Thus, Amarcand-ji performed his own funeral rites as he liberated his soul [7].

Although I am intrigued by fasting and enlightenment, I will try other ways to attain it. Come on. We only have one shot at life. There are no do-overs!

Complications and Death

Fasting could endanger a person's health and possibly result in a faster's death. The fasting does not cause death unless the faster has starved himself or herself. Otherwise, starting the feeding cycle causes problems, or the faster suffers from severe medical issues that fasting cannot heal and cure.

One of the most significant risks associated with prolonged fasts, particularly those lasting between 7 and 10 days, is the potential onset of Refeeding Syndrome [24]. This is a crucial point to consider, and it is why I strongly discourage extended fasts beyond two days, unless they are conducted under the supervision of a medical professional.

Our bodies rely on a diverse range of minerals such as calcium, chloride, magnesium, phosphorus, potassium, and sodium to support living tissues [11, 24]. When dissolved in water, these minerals form electrolytes that are crucial for various bodily functions. The water allows these suspended minerals to create charged particles, which are essential for many chemical reactions that sustain life. These electrolytes play a vital role in our overall health and well-being.

The body strictly balances the electrolytes during feeding and fasting [11]. However, a faster can experience Refeeding Syndrome as they start the feasting cycle. Refeeding syndrome comes from the digestive system's lack of minerals to break down food, as the digestive system steals minerals away from the blood and cells. A lack of minerals causes electrolyte imbalances. The imbalances cause heart arrhythmias, cardiac arrest, respiratory failure, seizures, or a host of other complications and problems [17, 24]. Symptoms can manifest themselves for up to a week [24].

People with anorexia, alcoholism, diabetes, cancer, or bowel disease are susceptible to refeeding syndrome [11]. These people are usually malnourished and underweight [11], and fasting creates a great shock to their bodies.

In the case of prolonged fasting, the body eventually transitions into a state of starvation. As the body depletes its fat reserves and absorbs noncritical tissues, the faster's hunger pangs return. If the faster chooses to continue abstaining, they enter a dangerous state of starvation. At this point, the body starts breaking down tissues and cells from vital organs for energy [3]. Simultaneously, the body's core temperature drops as it desperately tries to conserve energy [3, 14].

Dr. Shelton noted in a handful of cases when the faster could not eat food again [3]. After eating, the faster became sick and vomited the food. The inability to eat may stem from the refeeding syndrome. Subsequently, these fasters become starvation if they cannot kick-start the feasting cycle again.

Fasters who have fasted three days or more should transition to food by drinking juice and eating broths, fruits, or light soups. After extended fasts, the stomach lacks the enzymes to break down food. One YouTuber reported kidney failure after he ate a regular meal after a 20-day fast. Unfortunately, people show little symptoms of kidney or liver problems until 75% or more of the organ is destroyed and begins malfunctioning.

The faster suffers from an incurable disease, or the disease progressed to an advanced stage beyond fasting's curing range. Unfortunately, sick people resort to fasting as the last measure and not the first. If a disease such as cancer grows too large and spreads throughout the body, fasting will not heal the disease. In addition, patients taking harmful drugs and medicines for years also damage their bodies severely [9]. Unfortunately, fasting has its limits.

Fasting deaths, at last, occur rarely, but the deaths make front-page news. Even in the days of Dr. Shelton and Upton Sinclair, the newspapers widely reported fasting deaths [1, 3]. Dr. Shelton and Sinclair lamented that the authorities should conduct autopsies to thoroughly identify the correct cause of death because fasting unlikely caused the deaths. Most likely, another complication caused death. However, the reporters sensationalize fasting deaths to sell newspapers or capture a larger TV viewing audience.

The most notorious case of fasting comes from Linda Hazzard, the starvation doctor. She operated a fasting clinic in the early 1900s, and at least 15 people died at her fasting clinic. She was convicted of manslaughter in 1912 for the death of a wealthy British woman who weighed less than 50 pounds (or 22.7 kg) at the time of her death. Linda forged her signature on the British woman's will and stole the assets from her estate. The governor of the state of Washington pardoned her in 1916. Lastly, Linda Hazzard (1908, 1927) also wrote two fasting books, *Fasting for the Cure of Disease* and *Scientific Fasting: The Ancient and Modern Key to Health* [231, 232].

5. Types of Fasting

"A little starvation can really do more for the average sick man than can the best medicines and the best doctors."

– Mark Twain

Our bodies differ, and thus, our fasting regimes differ. For example, those with a mild hormone imbalance can make a simple dietary adjustment, like reducing sugar or eliminating gluten (for those with gluten sensitivity), that restores balance and alleviates health issues. We must explore and discover what methods work best for us, as what may be effective for one person may yield different results for another.

Exercise and diet modifications can also effectively rebalance hormones, as they introduce stress to the body. For some, this may be enough to restore hormonal equilibrium, eliminating the need for fasting. However, for those who require a more significant intervention, fasting can be considered as a last resort, a step beyond exercise and diet restriction.

We compare fasting to the Richter scale. Reducing our sugar intake shakes the body a little like an earth tremor. Diet restriction and exercise are small earthquakes. They both place stress on the body. A juice fast is a moderate earthquake, while intermittent fasting shakes the body like a major earthquake and rocks the body to its core. At last, a dry fast is a major earthquake and hurricane pummeling the body simultaneously. The dry fast places the most stress on the body as the fasters deprive themselves of food and fluids.

Before we discuss the types of fasts, we need to discuss people who should not fast. If the wrong people begin fasting, it could lead to health problems and possibly death.

Who Should Not Fast?

Fasting affects the body profoundly, such as lowering blood glucose and blood pressure [17, 31, 50, 51]. People taking insulin or high blood pressure medication can jeopardize their life. The insulin and high blood pressure medications could drop the blood sugar level and blood pressure to lethal levels [109]. Thus, we listen to our bodies. If our blood sugar levels drop too much, we could become irritable and hungry, feel nervous and nauseous, and experience shaking and sweating [11]; indicating hypoglycemia or low blood sugar. People with Type II diabetes keep a candy bar, a bottle of juice, or a sugary soda at hand in case their blood sugar level drops too much. Failure to raise blood sugar levels could result in death [11].

The following people should not fast, or they should fast under medical supervision.

> **Individuals with Severe Diseases** [35]: Fasting can have a profound, powerful impact on the body. It is important to note that fasting could potentially complicate individuals with serious illnesses.

> **Pregnant Women** [9, 11, 14, 35]: A pregnant woman needs a rich supply of nutrients, vitamins, and minerals to support the healthy growth of her baby [10, 11]. Fasting during pregnancy could potentially deprive the baby of these essential elements, leading to harm [11].

> **Breastfeeding Mothers** [11, 14]: The reason is identical to pregnant women. Women need abundant vitamins and minerals to produce nutrient-enriched breast milk to support the baby's growth [10, 11]. Also, a fast halts milk secretion [14].

> **Infants, Children, and Teenagers** [11, 35]: The bodies of infants, children, and teenagers grow rapidly. They need abundant nutrients, vitamins, and minerals to support their rapid growth. In some cases, doctors have fasted infants and young children to overcome serious viral infections or medical ailments [2, 3, 14]. For example, a two-year-old overcame polio by fasting for 47 days as his weight dropped from 32 pounds (or 14.5 kg) to 15 pounds (or 6.8 kg) [14].

- **Type 1 Diabetics** [9-11, 35, 109]: People with diabetes must monitor their glucose blood levels during a fast. They may have trouble maintaining normal glucose levels. Diabetes may cause large swings in blood sugar from too high to too low.

- **Kidney Problems** [9, 35]: Fasting stresses the kidneys as the kidneys filter the blood.

- **Liver Disease** [9]: Fasting stresses the liver.

- **People Suffering from Gastroesophageal Reflux Disease** [11]: For gastroesophageal reflux disease (GERD), the stomach acid flows upward into the esophagus. Then the acid burns and damages the esophagus [11]. Overweight or obese people can suffer from GERD because the abdominal fat constricts the stomach and pushes the stomach acids into the esophagus [11].

- **People Lacking MCAD:** Although rare, some people lack an enzyme called medium-chain acyl-CoA dehydrogenase (MCAD) [9]. The body needs this enzyme to oxidize fatty acids [9]. Thus, fasting is a risk for these individuals because they cannot consume fats for energy.

- **Severe Anemia** [9]: Anemia is a person with a red blood cell deficiency. Fasting amplifies the negative effects of anemia.

- **Advanced Stages of Cancer** [9]: Cancer has spread to different areas and organs of the body. The cancer patient has lost weight, stopped eating, and could be dehydrated. A fast could worsen these problems.

- **Acquired Immune Deficiency Syndrome (AIDS)** [9]: The HIV virus has demolished a person's immune system. The stress from fasting may be too great with a weakened immune system.

> **People with Toxic Levels of DDT Stored in Their Body Fat** [35]: This is unusual. The body tends to dump toxins into fat tissue during the feeding cycle. When fasters begin burning fat from their bodies, they release the toxins into their bodies again.

People afflicted with the following conditions can fast but require medical supervision. These medical conditions are less severe than the previous list.

> **People taking medications** [11]: Fasting lowers both insulin levels and blood pressure [9, 11, 12, 31, 37, 48, 50, 51, 120]. A person taking insulin during a fast can reduce blood sugar levels to lethal levels [11, 12]. Taking high blood pressure medication during a fast can drop blood pressure to dangerous levels. Low blood pressure causes light-headedness [11]. Also, fasting strengthens the potency and sensitivity of some medications [3, 14]. Please consult a medical doctor to adjust medications for fasting.

> **Gout:** The body retains excess uric acid in the blood instead of excreting the uric acid in the bladder. The uric acid forms crystals in the joints, causing arthritis and joint pain [11]. Fasting leads to a build of uric acid [11, 12, 17, 31, 51]. Fasters without gout can easily handle the increase in uric acid, but gout sufferers may not. Several medical doctors say that most people afflicted with gout experience no trouble fasting [9, 11, 137]. For example, in a study of prolonged fasting between 4 and 21 days, only one subject experienced gout out of 1,422 healthy participants [31].

> **Malnourished and Underweight People** [9-11, 109]: At the turn of the 20th century, some people suffered from malnutrition because their digestive systems could not process food efficiently. They fasted for a week or two, so their bodies repaired their digestive system [1-3, 9]. Then the malnourished people gained healthy weight as their bodies absorbed the

nutrients from the food during the feasting cycle [1-3, 9]. The worry is the dividing line between fasting and starvation since malnourished people lack the fat to endure long fasts.

We discuss fasting in the order in which it stresses the body. People must proceed at the lowest levels before starting the more advanced forms. The juice fast is the easiest. Intermittent fasting comes next. Finally, the extended fast is third, while the dry fast is the hardest and strongest.

The Juice Fast

The juice fast is technically not a fast because the person does not abstain from drinking juice. Instead, the faster drinks the juice to replace food. The juice fast includes eating fresh fruits and vegetables.

The Christians call the juice fast the Daniel fast from one of the books in the Old Testament (Daniel 1 [5]). King Nebuchadnezzar of Babylon captured Daniel and three other children from Judah. Daniel and his friends refused to eat meat and drink wine from the king's table (Daniel 1 [5]). Instead, they ate pulses, meaning beans, lentils, and peas. The Daniel diet or fast includes all-natural foods except for meat and wine.

Some claim three days of juice fasting equals one day of water fasting. This is a famous saying that we cannot back up with scientific evidence. Which measure could we use to substantiate this claim?

The juice fast poses the following three problems:

➢ **Problem #1:** Juicing fruit extracts the sugar and removes the fiber. A faster's body quickly absorbs the sugar and spikes the insulin level [9, 233]. Then the faster becomes hungry when the sugar level plummets. The fiber in fruit slows the sugar absorption [233].

➢ **Problem #2:** Drinking juice contains sugar and spikes insulin [9, 233]. The high insulin prevents the faster from switching to ketones for fuel. Remember, the nutrient sensors, mTOR and AMPK, are sensitive to insulin and amino acids.

➢ **Problem #3:** The juice fast prevents the faster from entering the protein-sparing state. Consequently, a fasting person loses more muscle mass and less fat than a water fast [9].

The juice fast became popular with celebrities in 2012 and has since withered. We should not be surprised that the juice diet causes people to always be hungry, especially if they drink the sugar from fruit [234]. Even Upton Sinclair complained that the fruit diet made him ravenously hungry and weaker [1].

In the Book of Daniel, Daniel and his friends became fairer and fatter in the flesh (Daniel 1 [5]). Remember, being chubby was a sign of health and living well in those days. Readers wanting more information on the Daniel Fast should visit https://ultimatedanielfast.com/.

Some people live by the health benefits of a juice fast. Juices are easy on the stomach and provide the body with many vitamins and minerals. Accordingly, the juice fast imparts some health benefits. In Asia, health retreats and resorts offer customers juice fast, but the resorts charge prices that compete with five-star hotels.

We do not need to juice fast to enjoy freshly squeezed juices, which are rich in vitamins, minerals, and antioxidants. We can enjoy fresh juices during our feasting cycles, especially if we eat atrocious diets. In Malaysia, many stores, restaurants, and cafeterias sell fresh juice. Two favorites include lime juice and Three Sours. Three Sours is a juice drink made from lime, lemon, and sour plum. Other excellent juices include carrots, oranges, pineapple, and apples.

➢ **Tip #9:** Investing in a juice machine may be wise. Fresh juice contains many vitamins, minerals, and antioxidants. Even if we do not juice fast, we can enjoy fresh juices during our feasting cycles.

Intermittent Fasting

Intermittent fasting, one of the most popular, is easy to implement. First, we write down our reasons to fast. We must stay focused when fasting starts changing our lives. For example, we see massive weight loss, or we start catching the eyes of the opposite sex; we are tempted to keep pushing that fasting duration for the wrong reasons. Compulsive, impulsive personalities could take fasting out of control. Therefore, we must be clear about why we fast and when we will start our feeding cycle again.

> ➤ **Tip #10:** Be clear about why we are fasting. We need to define our goals and what we hope to achieve.

Fasting can be a dangerous activity. We lose the desire to eat once we jump over the hunger hurdle. We have no problems continuing a fast for days or weeks. Consequently, we must be clear about when to end a fast.

I started fasting to improve my health, i.e., autophagy. My goal was never about losing weight or becoming an athlete. Those are the frosting and chocolate sprinkles on the doughnut. I ended many fasts when I felt great and could keep going. I would walk to the gym to weigh myself. If I had gained no weight from my atrocious diet, I ended my fast after 24 or 36 hours. My goal is not to push the fasting duration but to keep my body healthy.

The next decision is to choose how long and frequently we should fast. Like exercise, we start slowly. I first implemented a simple rule—no food or drink between 6 PM and 6 AM. We may drink water, tea, or coffee without sugar, honey, and milk.

> ➤ **Tip #11:** We should implement a daily 12-hour feeding window and a 12-hour fasting window.

We do not follow strict rules. If we meet friends for a Saturday night dinner or are invited to a party, by all means, we go and enjoy ourselves. Fasting is about living and enjoying life's little pleasures.

Violating the rule once a week will not hurt. I will not hesitate to end a fast prematurely if I am offered good food. I know I will fast twice weekly for the rest of my life. A day here and there of ending a fast early will matter little.

The next step in fasting is converting our bodies into fat-burning machines called fat adaptation. Many of us spent our lives being sugar burners. That means our bodies have not adapted to burning fat, which the body needs to enter a fasting state. It may be a good idea to start a high protein, low carbohydrate diet, such as the Adkins, South Beach, Zone, Protein Power, Sugar Busters, or the Stillman Diet. The Ketogenic Diet is also gaining popularity as a high-fat, moderate protein, and low-carbohydrate diet.

We use a diet temporarily to help our bodies transition towards burning fat for fuel.

> **Tip #12:** We should start a low-carbohydrate diet two weeks before our first fast to help our bodies transition into fat-burning machines.

Once our bodies become accustomed to burning fat and we have no trouble with a 12-hour fasting window, we just extend the fasting window. If we want to fast 15 hours, we delay eating breakfast by an additional three hours one day per week [10] or eat dinner three hours earlier once per week. It is that simple! Now, we are fasting for 15 hours once per week.

We utilize another trick to improve the fasting experience: We avoid foods high in sugar. If I eat cookies, ice cream, or doughnuts, I am ravenous again after two hours. We can save the cookies, ice cream, and doughnuts as a treat when we break the fast. Protein and fat fill our stomachs and make us feel satiated.

> **Tip #13:** Our last meal before the fast should be carbohydrate-free. The body burns carbohydrates quickly, causing insulin levels to peak and crash. The crash awakens hunger pangs.

When I first started fasting, I did an 18-hour fast once a week. The first couple of times, I thought I would die. Fasting is both physiological and psychological. The low-carbohydrate diet helps with the physiological part. Once fasting becomes routine, we must learn to overcome the mental hurdle.

The psychological hurdle is difficult. Sometimes, I felt hungry during a fast, but I learned to persist and not eat. When I started the 24-hour fasts, the 20-hour mark became dangerous. I would walk around the mall like a zombie, smelling the freshly baked cookies and the cheese sizzling on a baked pizza. I just wanted to eat even when I was not hungry. We conditioned ourselves to eat at least three times a day since birth. Thus, we must rewire our brains to escape the desire to eat food.

The first several fasts will be difficult. We may need a crutch when we start fasting. It feels weird to go for an extended time without eating. I ate some hard-boiled eggs with hot sauce during the first several fasts. Technically, I violated the fast and introduced protein into my body. If the crutch turns into a meal, we do not worry about it. We enjoy our meal. We can start fasting on another day.

> **Tip #14:** In the beginning, we need a crutch to help us endure the fast. We can eat a low-carbohydrate snack. The Keto Diet offers many good, low-carbohydrate snacks, such as chicken, cheese, nuts, or berries. Once fasting becomes second nature, we drop the crutch and eliminate all snacks.

We continue fasting until it becomes routine. When we need to expand our fast, we start fasting twice weekly. We must spread our fasts over the week between two full days of feeding. For example, it felt so natural to fast; I started fasting twice weekly without thinking about it. After two days of feasting, I did not feel hungry again on the third day.

I accidentally came across a good rule. I maintain a ratio of 1 to 2 for fasting and feasting cycles. For example, if I fast for one day, I feed for the next two days. The first day of feeding sometimes throws my body out of equilibrium, but then everything turns to normal for the second feeding day. We also must ensure we eat enough food to provide our bodies with the necessary nutrients.

> ➤ **Tip #15:** Maintain a ratio of 1 to 2 for fasting and feasting cycles. If we fast for three days, we should feast for six days before starting the next fast. We must ensure our bodies obtain the minimum nutritional requirements.

After several weeks, we can extend the duration of our fasting if we need to. However, we must check ourselves and ask ourselves why we are fasting. If we want to hasten the pace of our weight loss, there may be better ideas than extending the fast. It took me thirty years to pack 35 pounds (or 15.9 kg) of fat. I am more than happy that fasting removed this fat within a year. My goal is not to lose this weight in one month. My fasting goal is to improve my health and fast intermittently for the rest of my life. We use fasting to make our bodies healthy. Then our body decides how much fat we should carry.

We can boost our fasting duration by 3—or 6-hour increments. I started with 18-hour fasts once weekly, then fasted twice weekly, then 24-hour fasts, and then 30-hour fasts. I am going for the weekly super cleanse, a 48-hour fast once weekly. I fast beyond 24 hours because I feel and see the health benefits and believe I am prolonging my life.

We must drink plenty of fluids during a fast because fasting dehydrates the body [9]. Food contains water, so since we stop eating, we need to drink extra fluids to make up for the shortfall. Chapter 6 discusses the permitted fasting drinks.

> ➤ **Tip #16:** Drink plenty of water [1, 9, 10]. Since fasters stop eating, they must drink more water to compensate for the water deficit. We could burn additional calories by drinking cold water since our bodies must warm the water to body temperature [235].

Fasting subjects the body to stress. When we have just started fasting, we should take it easy. We should rest, relax, and not exercise. If the fasting euphoria makes us spacey, we should avoid driving a vehicle or using power tools. Once we become accustomed to fasting, we can resume our usual activities.

> **Tip #17:** When we start fasting, we should take it easy for the first several fasts. We can exercise once our bodies have adapted to fasting [134].

Sometimes, we should fast back to back to avoid weight gain during celebrations or when we become sick. For example, Malaysians celebrate Christmas, Chinese New Year, the feasting celebrations after Ramadan, and Gawai, the harvest celebration of the Borneo tribes. This is a perfect time to eat delicious ethnic food. Fasting is about living and enjoying life, and I love eating. I did not become obese because I didn't like food.

The Borneo tribes celebrate the season's harvest, Gawai, a time when everyone eats and drinks. For Gawai in 2018, I ate and drank all day as we visited a half-dozen houses on Friday. The hosts offered a well-stocked buffet of delicious foods, such as curry chicken, beef rendang, prawn crackers with peanuts and anchovies, and sliced tropical fruits. The Borneo natives believe in drinking copious amounts of homemade rice wine and whiskeys of questionable grades and qualities.

Afterward, I fasted for 18 hours and then had lunch at Pizza Hut and KFC. Then I fasted another 18 hours. I neither gained nor lost weight, so I was not nervous when I headed to the gym and stepped on the weight scales.

> **Tip #18:** We employ back-to-back fasts to prevent weight gain from celebrations and holidays. These are special occasions that we should enjoy and cherish. Accordingly, we apply back-to-back fasts once in a while for weight maintenance.

It sounds like I contradicted myself. As I already stated, I do not fast for weight loss. However, I do alter my fasting schedule to prevent weight gain.

Fasting contains a psychological part. We conditioned ourselves to eat food at least three times daily since birth. Breaking this habit is difficult. Often, we may feel hungry during a fast, but the hunger pangs come in waves. We learn to endure the hunger waves and keep fasting. Each time we fast, pushing the fasting duration becomes easier and easier.

> **Tip #19:** We learn to endure hunger pangs. One trick is to stay busy and keep our minds focused on non-food activities. We can also join fasting groups on social media, such as Facebook, to find mutual support and fasting buddies.

Fasting has another benefit. We can utilize fasting to identify food allergies. For example, we suspect we are allergic or sensitive to gluten. If we have fasted for at least 15 hours, we have cleared the food from our digestive system. Subsequently, we can eat a slice of bread or pastry and note how we react. However, this technique only works for fasts of two days or fewer because extended fasts require an adjustment period to consume food again.

> **Tip #20:** We can utilize short fasts between 15 and 48 hours to identify food allergies.

If we feel nauseous, dizzy, fatigued, or lethargic, and the symptoms do not go away, we end the fast [11]. Our health is more important than the time we spend in a fast. Thus, we will live another day too fast in the future.

> **Tip #21:** We end the fast if we feel ill, dizzy, fatigued, or lethargic, and these side effects do not subside. We can live another day and start another fast.

Intermittent fasting is flexible and easily fits into anyone's lifestyle. We can adjust the fasting schedule to fit into our busy lives. I prefer to fast on Mondays and Fridays on my workdays and leave my weekends open for food and friends. I also fast by the clock. For example, I eat breakfast after 6 AM, lunch before 12, and dinner before 6 PM I have no trouble keeping track of my fast since I go in 6-hour increments.

> **Tip #22:** We can easily track our fasts if we eat at 6 AM, noon, and 6 PM Then we work with either 3—or 6-hour increments.

We can also download free fasting trackers for our smartphones. The trackers store a log of our fasts.

When we fast, we should avoid people. Fasters become more sensitive to other people's emotions. I lose patience and become irritable and grumpy. This is not a good time to interact with people. I refused to believe I was grumpy, but my best friend could tell when I was fasting, i.e., I was grumpier.

> **Tip #23:** We should avoid people when fasting because we become hypersensitive to other people's emotions [29]. Furthermore, prolonged fasts tend to make fasters angry [236].

Fasters should be warned about one potential drawback to fasting. A faster may experience a ghost infection when a past chronic infection returns during a fast. Dr. Moser called this retracing [29]. I suffered from a chronic ear infection that periodically returned. During my first several fasts, the ear infection returned and disappeared quickly. Nevertheless, I never suffered an ear infection again. Other fasters have reported ghost injuries where previous, old injuries started to hurt again.

> **Tip #24:** Fasters may relive a ghost infection or a ghost pain if they suffered from a chronic, reoccurring infection or an old injury in the past. Just keep warm and drink plenty of fluids.

Fasting has other benefits. I travel often and balk at the high prices at international airports. The food is overpriced and guaranteed to give travelers diarrhea. Once, I felt robbed at the Guangzhou Baiyun International Airport in China when I paid $30 for a $2 bowl of Ramen noodles. Embarking on a long trip is an excellent time to start fasting, which leads to the next tip.

> **Tip #25:** When we start a long trip, that is the perfect time to start a fast. Thus, we avoid expensive, substandard food that gives us the traveler's diarrhea and digestion problems.

After six months of intermittent fasting, I experimented and tried different things. For example, I started a fast with a bag of Oreo cookies, dipping milk, and a sweet coffee for lunch. That was a terrible idea. I had one incredible sugar buzz for the first three hours of the fast. Then I felt queasy and dizzy until the fifth hour. After the fifth hour, it was smooth sailing, and I ended the fast 30 hours later. I become so well adapted to intermittent fasting; a crazy, sugary meal could not stop me from fasting. It has become second nature.

I tried to get my Malaysian Chinese girlfriend, Alice, to fast. I bribed her with 100 Malaysian ringgits (or $25) to fast one weekend for 18 hours. One hundred ringgits is more like $50 because of the low Malaysian prices. For instance, I can get an excellent lunch of two pieces of curry chicken, rice, and herbal tea for 12 ringgits (or $3) at a Chinese cafe. Alice did all right and made it to 16 hours. Unfortunately, she found a bag of Skittles under the car seat and gorged herself, thus breaking the fast. I tried to get her to fast on other occasions and upped the bribe to 200 ringgits (or $50). No luck! She refuses to fast. She believes food gives her energy. No food – no energy.

The significance is the Chinese place a high priority on money. For example, I had several dates with Chinese women that felt more like job interviews. On one date, I received three hours of financial advice and tips. My date even estimated the cash flows and profits at the restaurant where we dined. Of course, the date was a bargain since a three-hour consultation with a financial advisor would cost some serious money. (These were okay dates, but I had some crazy dates in Asia.) Hence, Alice turning down the money for a simple task means she loves eating food too much.

I tried to get Alice to fast for two reasons. First, I wanted her to experience the health benefits, and she could start fasting independently. She usually goes on diets to lose weight, which has a high failure rate. Second, I wanted to get information about women fasting because a female blogger on YouTube suggested some women have trouble fasting. The female blogger claimed that women who skip meals without difficulties can easily fast while others experience troubles. For example, in one study, healthy men became more sensitive to insulin after a 36-hour fast than women [30]. In another study, overweight women who fasted became less sensitive to insulin compared to the diet-restricted control group [126]. Insulin insensitivity may be the women's bodies ensuring the brain has access to glucose, preventing other cells, tissues, and organs from using this glucose [139]. Thus, fasting impacts men and women differently.

I am also curious whether Alice could fast since she is a sugar addict. On several occasions, I sipped her Starbucks drink and winced over the extreme sweetness. I wonder if I am more surprised that a barista can pack a ton of sugar molecules into a dense liquid or that Alice can quickly drink her overly sweet concoction.

The Prolonged Fast

Any fasts extending beyond 24 hours are prolonged because the fast stretches for two or more days. The 24 hours is an artificial construction, but researchers have noted "adverse" changes in healthy men's mitochondria, the cells' energy furnace, after a 24-hour fast [13]. In addition, I believe fasts beyond 24 hours help prolong longevity, but no studies have shown this in humans. Rodent studies back prolonged fasts for extending lifespans. However, a 24-hour fast shocks rodents' bodies greatly because of their greater metabolism.

Fasting beyond two days forces the faster into dangerous territory. My longest fast lasted 50 hours. I experienced no hunger, discomfort, or medical complications when I broke my fast. I could have easily fasted for another day if I had wanted to. Nevertheless, my fasting goal is to get health benefits via autophagy, apoptosis of senescent cells, and activating the longevity genes.

Some people must fast beyond 24 hours because they need a shock to their bodies. Some people, including me, have insulin resistance. Not only does the body produce too much insulin, but the insulin levels also remain persistently high even when the digestive system ceases food processing [12]. Consequently, persistently high insulin levels keep the body in fat storage mode and prevent our bodies from burning fat reserves [12].

Fasting, accordingly, helps reset insulin and other hormones such as ghrelin. Ghrelin sends a satiation signal that we should stop eating [12, 143, 237]. When our bodies screw up this hormone, we can be highly overweight and always feel that we are starving. When I was obese, I always felt hungry and wanted to snack every two hours.

Researchers argue that ghrelin does not provide a satiation signal [237]. Instead, the hormone prepares the digestive system to anticipate food [237]. Scientists and doctors have identified many hormones involved in satiety and hunger signals. They are searching for the magic pill that would help dieters lose weight without the hunger pangs.

Fasting restores the satiety and hunger signals by shocking and stressing the body. For example, some electronic gadgets like a computer start malfunctioning. We must turn off the device to reset it. Some devices need to remain off for several minutes. Fasting does the same to our hormones. We turn off the digestive system for a while, which brings the persistently high insulin levels down and resets the sensitivity of our hormones, such as ghrelin [37]. Fasting is resetting our hormones.

Of course, I do not fast beyond 48 hours because I reap all the health benefits of fasting. For example, if autophagy switches on after 16 hours of abstaining from food and I fast twice a week for 24 hours, then in one year, I fasted 104 days. However, each fast has 16 hours without autophagy. If I deduct the 16 hours from each fast, I fasted for 34.7 days with autophagy. Fantastic! I spent over one month in autophagy yearly! (Please note that many researchers and bloggers debate when autophagy kicks in, but the mTOR sensor and AMPK are mechanisms to control autophagy that we discussed in Chapter 2).

We should only last up to 48 hours for people wanting to practice prolonged fasts. I list several reasons why we should end the fast within two days.

➢ **Stabilize Weight:** People would fast for 21 days or more in the old days. They would lose 21 pounds (or 9.5 kg). Then they continued their same lifestyle after the fast and regained the weight. In one study, 50% of the fasters regained their weight on a 14-day fast, while 24% of the subjects continued to lose weight [137]. On the other hand, 43% of fasters who were obese could maintain a lower weight by fasting intermittently, while 17% continued losing weight [21]. That success rate of fasting squashes the one percent success rate of calorie restriction.

Medical doctors warn of the dangers of yo-yo dieting, in which a person loses weight and then regains it. Thus, we should fast intermittently every week to stabilize our weight and smooth the fluctuations.

> **Metabolism:** Fasting beyond two days reduces a faster's metabolism [23]. That is the trick. We fast for one day or two days. Then we eat well during our feasting cycle to keep that metabolism roaring and devouring energy. Short fasts do not slow metabolism [49] and may even boost metabolism by 3% [23].

> **Refeeding Syndrome:** Extended fasts between 7 and 10 days may result in refeeding syndrome [24].

Refeeding syndrome occurs when the faster or starving person starts eating food again, and the food throws the person's electrolytes out of balance. Electrolytes are salts such as magnesium, phosphate, potassium, and sodium dissolved in water and are critical to chemical reactions to sustain life [11, 24]. Severe electrolyte imbalances cause heart arrhythmia, respiratory failure, dementia, seizures, and a host of other symptoms and problems [24]. Two-day fasts or less reduce the complications of refeeding syndrome.

> **Maximize Fat Burning:** Fasts between 18 and 24 hours are sufficient for the body to break down fats and triglycerides [125]. Thus, fasters are burning some of their fat stores.

➢ **Effective Weight Loss:** In one study, healthy subjects increased their caloric intake by 30% for the first meal after a 36-hour fast with a preference for more fatty foods [238]. After the first meal, they resumed their standard eating patterns [238]. Thus, subjects still lost weight because they failed to make up for the deficient calories they missed while on a fast. (In this regard, fasting corresponds to calorie restriction because fasters are reducing their total calories).

Some people fast for three days because they believe the body renews the immune system. In a mice study, a prolonged fast of at least three days caused the mice's bodies to remove the poorly functioning, old white cells [239]. (The study used the fasting-mimicking diet that permits limited food consumption during the fast [239]). Unfortunately, our bodies are complex, and white blood cells come in two broad classes: Lymphocytes and phagocytes. Lymphocytes adapt to new threats, including T, B, and natural killer cells. The T cells cause apoptosis of virus-infected cells like a tack popping a balloon; B cells produce antibodies to destroy foreign invaders, while natural killer cells obliterate cancerous cells. On the other hand, phagocytes resemble Pac-Man and gobble foreign invaders, dead cells, and cell debris. During the feasting cycle, our bodies quickly regenerate the white blood cells [239]. Thus, prolonged fasters have new, efficient immune systems to defend their bodies against foreign invaders.

People who fast for three days or more should eat light food to slowly re-introduce food into their digestive system. The stomach lacks the enzymes to break down the food. Fasters should drink freshly squeezed juice or bone broth for their first meal and add steamed vegetables for the next meal [1, 9, 28, 240]. Dr. Shelton recommended fasters drink fresh fruit juice every two hours on the first meal day and three meals of fruit the next day [3]. The Soviet doctors and Upton Sinclair added dairy products to the diet [1, 28]. However, Upton Sinclair (1911) admitted having trouble taking dairy products after an extended fast. In addition, some people doing extended water fasts follow the fast with the juice fast or Daniel diet. Fasters should avoid salt, pepper, and spices until their stomachs can handle them [9]. At last, the Soviet doctors advised patients to avoid meat for some time [28]. Meanwhile, Dr. Shelton recommended eating plenty of protein to allow the body to rebuild structures lost from autophagy and cell death (apoptosis) [3].

As fasters start their feasting cycle, they may experience diarrhea. Thus, we must be careful when passing gas after our first meal or carrying clean underwear. I occasionally experienced diarrhea after completing fasts beyond 24 hours. When I break a fast, I get diarrhea. Boy, is it nasty? My body is finding nasty things to remove. Of course, I will wait to see if the problem is corrected before taking Imodium. Most of the time, the problem corrects itself before the next meal.

I could not find why the diarrhea occurs, but I have a theory of why this diarrhea is so foul. Our liver filters the blood during a fast and removes debris and old blood cells. Remember – the liver has no food to process so that it can work on other things. Then the liver passes the debris through the gallbladder and into the small intestines. The body purges itself of this foulness from the small intestines into the colon and out of the body. Now, we see why the hygienists performed regular enemas at the fasting clinics.

Even though I do not recommend fasts beyond two days, some people require prolonged fasts. For example, fasting to reduce the size of tumors requires two weeks or more [3, 9]. Dr. Shelton fasted patients between three days and two months [3]. He supervised six fasts beyond 60 days, with his longest fast of 90 days.

People with medical conditions must fast under a doctor's supervision at a fasting clinic. The clinic staff can monitor blood pressure, glucose blood level, and electrolytes while the doctors adjust medications as needed [9]. Then the doctors terminate the fast to prevent endangering a patient's health and life.

The Dry Fast

The dry fast, also called the absolute fast, is the strongest fast. The faster abstains from all food and drink for some time. Some claim that one day of dry fasting equals three days of a water fast. This claim is more of a statement because which measure could we use to support it? Some advocates claim the dry fast is a virus killer, which induces three times the autophagy of water fast. Research still needs to validate these claims.

I, nevertheless, found a weight loss ratio of 1 to 3 between water and dry fasts. For example, on a dry fast, research subjects lost 3 pounds (or 1.39 kg) daily [3, 240]. Meanwhile, a person loses about a pound (or 0.45 kg) daily on a water fast [3, 9, 14], which gives a one-to-three ratio. The researchers do not answer whether the higher weight loss comes from water loss. Otherwise, the fasters would quickly regain the water weight once they started eating and drinking again.

Water loss is the mechanism that intensifies the fast. The water loss increases the salts in the blood, such as sodium, and sodium draws water out of the cells [241]. With less water, the cells shrink. This stresses the cells because each cell has a micro-tube network called microtubules that crisscross the cell like I-beams in a building. These microtubules maintain and support the cell structure. The dehydration also triggers autophagy that reorganizes the microtubules [68]. A shrinking cell concentrates proteins and could create misfolded proteins, which induce apoptosis, i.e., cell death [241]. The dry fast is stronger than water fast as autophagy reorganizes a cell's structure and removes damaged parts and misfolded proteins.

The dry fast comes as soft and hard dry fasts. The soft, dry fast allows fasters to brush their teeth, take showers, and wash their hands after using the bathroom. Meanwhile, fasters cannot even touch water during a hard, dry fast because their bodies absorb water through the skin during showers and brushing their teeth. Of course, we can use the dry fast to get out of house chores like washing the car or dishes.

The dry fast places more stress on the body than a water fast. The faster could become dehydrated quickly. The faster should not exercise or stand outside on a hot day since the body loses water from sweating. Furthermore, I moved to Southern Nevada in 2022. When I walked outside, the sun blasted its rays upon me during the summer. I became extremely thirsty walking to the store a block away. I had trouble doing dry fasts since the Nevadan climate is arid. I noticed my water fasts are much stronger there, too. Technically, Las Vegas is in the middle of the desert. That may explain why Jesus went into the desert too fast for 40 days.

When deprived of water, the body produces small quantities of water. For instance, the body produces 107 grams of water from 100 grams of fat [242], which equals about 0.34 liter for 24 hours of dry fasting. (The calculation assumes a person burns 2,500 fat calories during one day). Some estimates claim the body produces about one quart (or liter) of water daily, which is triple the previous estimate. Of course, the body also conserves water as water becomes scarce.

Some fasters claim the dry fast is the easiest to practice. Drinking fluids awakens hunger in some people during a water fast. People who want to experiment with the dry fast must follow the following six rules.

> **Rule 1:** The faster it is clear why he or she uses a dry fast. If we dry fast, we should take it easy, stay in bed, cover ourselves with a blanket, and relax. This is the perfect time to catch up on our favorite TV shows or read a good book. Fresh air, rest, and sunshine are also good for the body.

> **Rule 2:** The person is an experienced faster. Fasting resembles exercise. The more a person fasts, the easier fasting gets. The body quickly adapts to frequent fasts. Thus, fasters have completed many water fasts before attempting the dry fast.

> **Rule 3:** The dry fast is not an extended fast. We should ignore the YouTubers who dry fast for three days or longer. They always post a disclaimer at the beginning of their videos for entertainment purposes only. The dry fast dehydrates the body

and jeopardizes a faster's health and life. In a study, healthy subjects experienced no health problems during a five-day, dry fast [240]. Of course, I dry fast at least twice a month for 24 hours. The body quickly adapts, and the dry fast becomes easy except in the dry climate of Southern Nevada.

> **Rule 4:** We should not exercise or be outside in hot weather. The dry fast dehydrates the body, which jeopardizes health in hot weather. Athletic performance also declines during a dry fast [243], so dry fasting may be the wrong time to train for competitions. The lower athletic performance comes from dehydration and poor sleep, as Muslims awaken early to eat breakfast before dawn [243]. Thus, the muscles store less glycogen from the carbs that the muscles utilize for energy.

> **Rule 5:** Heavy coffee and tea drinkers should be careful during a dry fast. They may experience headaches and mood swings since they suffer from caffeine withdrawal symptoms during a fast [242]. Fasters may need to abstain from coffee and tea for several days to ease withdrawal symptoms [242].

> **Rule 6:** People with eye diseases should avoid a dry fast [242]. A dry fast exacerbates the symptoms of cataracts, dry eye syndrome, or glaucoma [242].

Dehydrated fasters experience increased thirst, dark or more yellow urine than usual, headache, sleepiness, or dizziness, or a combination of two or more symptoms [244]. Fasters must end the dry fast and drink fluids when fasting becomes uncomfortable.

The Muslims practice dry fasting. During the month of Ramadan, Muslims cannot eat or drink anything from sunrise to sunset nor partake in sensual pleasures as they fast to commune with God [245]. Islam exempts people who are vulnerable to dry fasting, such as children, the elderly, pregnant women, breastfeeding women, women during their menstrual cycle, and severely sick people [245].

Muslims limit the duration of a dry fast from sunrise to sunset. If Ramadan falls in June, the longest day occurs during the summer solstice, around June 20 in the northern hemisphere. The day lasts 17 hours. Consequently, Muslims fast between 11 and 22 hours, depending on where they live on the earth [84]. Therefore, Muslims would never dry fast beyond 24 hours unless they lived in the North Pole with the midnight sun.

I lived in Malaysia and conversed with the Muslims about fasting. The Muslims are surprised when I tell them I fast intermittently. They concede that dry fasting imparts many health benefits as they fast during Ramadan, but they avoid fasting every Monday and Thursday per week. Remember, Islamic law requires all eligible Muslims to fast during Ramadan, but Muslims can volunteer to intermittent fast twice weekly. Again, when people feel obligated or forced into fasting, they never want to fast voluntarily.

We need more evidence of whether a 12-hour fast is long enough despite the dry fast being stronger than the water fast. Both healthy males and females experienced drops in LDL cholesterol, blood glucose level, insulin growth factor, and inflammation markers [33, 84, 105, 245]. Meanwhile, women exhibited increased HDL cholesterol, while the men lost weight and lowered triglycerides. I talked to one Muslim woman who is overweight and suffers from gout. Doctors treated her with chemotherapy for a brain tumor. She fasts regularly between sunrise and sunset and concedes that she feels much better when fasting but has lost no weight. She fasts about 12 hours regularly, which may need to be more. That leads to our next tip.

> **Tip #26:** Fasters may extend a dry fast or switch to water fast after sunset to boost the health benefits of fasting. Fasters can also embed a dry fast into a water fast by dry fasting for 24 hours and then switch to a water fast for 12 hours.

People should fast for at least 16 hours to attain the maximum benefits of fasting [143]. Depending on the person, fasting causes significant physiological changes between 12 and 16 hours into a fast. Both glycogen and insulin drop to new, lower plateaus after 12 hours after the last meal, while blood glucose sets to a lower level after 13 hours [53]. Glucagon, the opposing insulin hormone, peaks 13 hours into a fast [53]. The pancreas produces glucagon to message the muscles to release all glycogen and increases the fatty acids in the blood. Finally, the body begins breaking down fat into free fatty acids while the liver converts the free fatty acids into ketones. Thus, people must fast for at least 16 hours to switch their bodies from sugar-burning to fat-burning.

I tried the 24-hour dry fast. This was a perfect opportunity to catch up on Supernatural and the Winchester boys. The fast's euphoria returned after 8 hours into the fast. I haven't experienced euphoria in years on a water fast. I must water fast beyond 30 hours to get some remnants of euphoria.

During the dry fast, I alternated between shivering and being cold and sweating and being hot. I felt little pinpricks at different places on my body. I would feel a light pinprick on the right wrist, then on my ankle, and later on, on my left chest and other places on the body.

I used a soft dry fast, so I still took a shower, brushed my teeth, and washed my hands after using the bathroom—there was no need to make others suffer my stench and germs during a dry fast. I still urinated five times during the fast. However, I peed less frequently as the fast progressed, and the urine turned a darker yellow. Finally, I was surprised my mouth still produced saliva and felt good.

I experienced insomnia as I slept for four hours. I woke up at 2 AM and could not return to sleep. I did not feel refreshed entirely, but I did not feel terrible either. Nevertheless, I slept better on my following dry fasts. Now, the dry fasts have become routine.

I measured my weight during my first dry fast and lost 4.4 pounds (or 2 kg). Of course, I mainly lost water because 4.4 pounds of fat would translate into 15,500 calories. No way did I lose that much body fat within 24 hours! That is easily five days of food for me.

I ended the fast after 23 hours by drinking unsweetened strawberry tea. A half-hour later, I followed the tea with homemade cinnamon oatmeal bread with real butter. Perhaps it wasn't smart to make homemade bread and fill the house with a wonderful cinnamon, baking bread smell after not eating or drinking for 22 hours. The next night, I slept nine hours and woke up refreshed and ready to go.

I, consequently, incorporated at least two soft, dry fasts into my monthly intermittent fasting regimen. The dry fast is stronger, so hopefully, the dry fast imparts more health benefits to the body. Only time will tell. However, my body quickly adapted to dry fasting as the dry fast became just as easy as a water fast. Now, I almost feel no difference between feasting and a dry fast. The dry fast has become routine and monotonous except after exercising. Once, I tried to start a 24-hour dry fast after running for 45 minutes. I became severely dehydrated and had to drink unsweetened tea 18 hours into the fast.

Hormesis

The human body is a beautiful machine that adapts quickly to the environment, so mild stress strengthens the body, while severe stress damages it. We call this mild stress hormesis. For example, a short fast strengthens the body and imparts many health benefits. However, if we keep extending the duration of the fast, then the fast may place too much stress on the body and thus weaken it.

The key is to find the level of stress that strengthens the body the most. We regularly witness hormesis in the following ways.

➤ All drugs and medicines have a hormetic effect on the body. The substances benefit the body at low doses, but the substances become lethal at high doses. For example, a cup of coffee contains about 100 milligrams (or 0.1 grams) of caffeine. However, 20 grams of caffeine becomes lethal. That is about 100 cups of coffee. Nevertheless, people develop a tolerance to caffeine as they drink coffee regularly. Thus, they need higher doses of caffeine to get the same effect.

➤ Running is an excellent exercise for the body. The stress of running strengthens the lungs and circulatory system as the muscles demand oxygen to do work. However, just observe marathon runners. Some look sickly thin and emaciated because they impose too much stress on the body. Ironically, no one discusses the origin of the marathon. The Greek soldier Pheidippides ran 26 miles (42 kilometers) to Athens to report the victory of the Battle of Marathon. Then he collapsed and died from exhaustion.

➤ Animals and plants do not want to be eaten, so they develop defenses against predators. Animals can run or fight, whereas plants produce natural pesticides to sicken the predator with toxic chemicals [223]. We already discussed natural pesticides in fruits and vegetables in Chapter 4. We eat various foods to strengthen the body, but eating the same foods regularly may cause health problems as we constantly expose our bodies to the same poisons.

The critical point to hormesis is that the body adapts to the mild stress. Siim Land provides a good rule: We should continuously cycle through different regimes and conditions to strengthen the body [56]. Several examples include:

➤ We should alter the durations of our fasts. For instance, we water fast for 30 hours. Then our next fast lasts 18 hours. Then we fast for 25 hours. Perhaps we dry fast one time, and then water fasts the next. Once every couple of months, we do a prolonged three-day fast. The mix of short and long-duration fasts helps reduce diseases and contribute to longevity [246], preventing our bodies from adapting to the same fasts.

➤ We know the body's cells prefer glucose, i.e., sugar, to fats. However, most cells in the body can utilize ketones and fatty acids for fuel. (Remember, the liver, red blood, and 25% of the brain cells still need glucose). Some people fast and follow the ketogenic diet to remain in ketosis, whereas their bodies are constantly burning fat for fuel. The body may benefit more by cycling between standard and ketogenic diets as we continuously change the cells' energy source [65].

Of course, we know the converse is true – it is not always good to eat and burn carbohydrates for energy all the time. Hence, periodically abstaining from food can do wonders for the body.

6. Fasting Friendly Drinks and Supplements

"In anything, there has to be that moment of fasting, really, in order to enjoy the feast."

– Stephen Hough

In this chapter, we discuss drinks and supplements fasters can enjoy without breaking their fasts. For a true fast, a person abstains from food and drinks except water. However, the fasting person has many options for non-caloric beverages. The beverages must be free from sugar since sugar triggers an insulin response and forces the body out of the fasting state. Sugar comes in many disguises.

➤ Sugar includes table sugar, honey, and agave nectar [11].

➤ Sugar has many scientific names depending on the source: Fruits and honey (fructose), milk and dairy products (galactose and lactose), barley (maltose), and wood and straw (xylose).

➤ The food industry manufactures high fructose corn syrup from cornstarch. Technically, fructose may elicit a slight insulin response. The body's cells cannot use fructose directly for energy; the liver must convert it into fat.

The faster should avoid sugar substitutes such as aspartame, saccharin, and sucralose. The chemical industry manufactures sugar substitutes from artificial chemicals. We fasters should avoid artificial sugars since they can awaken hunger, which would cause us to end the fast prematurely. Furthermore, we must determine whether artificial sweeteners illicit an insulin response because of many conflicting studies [12]. On the other hand, stevia comes naturally from the plant *Stevia rebaudiana*. However, we do not know if stevia elicits an insulin response.

Many people consume zero-calorie drinks and sodas. However, drinking zero-calorie drinks may not reduce calories and provide little benefit in weight loss. In one study, 30 healthy males consumed a sugary strawberry-flavored beverage spiked with table sugar, aspartame, stevia, or monk fruit [247]. Monk fruit is a natural zero-calorie sweetener that is becoming popular among dieters. The participants showed no difference in calories consumed, blood sugar, and insulin spikes after eating [247]. Thus, we should avoid consuming drinks with artificial sugars since eating more food would make up for the zero calories.

Fasters can drink broth, coffee, flavored water, tea, soda water, and minerals and not violate their fast. Although these drinks have a touch of calories, the calories are not enough to kick the faster out of the fasting state. It is like a speeder slowing down over a speed bump to protect a car's suspension. Once the speeder crosses the speed bump, he or she returns to violating all the traffic laws again in full force.

Broth

Some fasters drink bone broth made from beef, pork, chicken, or fish bones. Bone broth contains traces of protein, fat, and carbohydrates [248]. People fasting for less than 24 hours may want to avoid bone broth since the protein and carbohydrates can halt the fasting state. A 0.42 cup (or 100 milliliters) of bone broth has 51 calories with trace elements and minerals such as calcium, magnesium, phosphorus, potassium, and sodium [11, 248]. Since the fasters eat some food, they can endure longer fasts [11]. The bone broth provides the body with essential electrolytes that help to avoid the refeeding syndrome when fasters kick-start their feeding cycles again [11].

> ➤ **Tip #27**—Bone Broth: Clean half a pound (or ¼ kg) of your favorite bones, such as beef, chicken, lamb, or pork. Simmer the bones in a covered water or crock pot with two bay leaves for at least four hours. Add sea or Himalayan salt and pepper during the last hour for taste. Sea and Himalayan salt contain trace elements and minerals. Add water as necessary to make at least four mugs of broth—refrigerate and reheat as needed.

Some recipes add vegetables to the broth. The vegetables add vitamins and minerals to the broth and carbohydrates. Thus, fasters beware.

Some medical experts recommend that fasters avoid bouillon cubes because they contain artificial flavors, colors, and monosodium glutamate [11]. However, they are convenient. Just drop a bouillon cube into a mug of hot water and enjoy.

An excellent choice is bouillon, Tom Yam, a spicy, sour Thai soup. The soup base comes from chicken or seafood stock, lemongrass, lime leaves, lime juice, fresh ginger, spicy chilies, fish sauce, brown sugar, and red curry paste. It packs a spicy punch but only adds 20 calories.

The salt has the potential to dehydrate faster. The body must muster extra water to expel excess salt in the urine. That is why we fasters should always drink plenty of fluids during a fast.

Coffee

Fasters who love their morning cup of joe can still enjoy their coffee as long as they add no sugar, cream, or milk. Sugar, cream, or milk could halt the fasting state in large quantities. In addition, dairy products contain lactose, both a sugar and a protein.

Black coffee is great when we get used to the taste. I lived in a tropical climate, so coffee on the rocks added a nice touch to my mornings. One teaspoon of instant coffee contains four calories, trace levels of minerals such as calcium, magnesium, phosphorus, and potassium, and a small quantity of niacin [248]. The coffee's nutrients depend on the coffee bean's origin, type, roasting, and manufacturer.

➤ **Tip #28**—Cold Brew Coffee: We become tired of the bitter taste of some coffees. Adding three tablespoons of ground coffee to a small water bottle to make our iced black coffee is a refreshing solution. Shake and refrigerate for several days. Then filter the coffee, add ice, and voila! We have a delicious cold brew that weakens the bitterness of strong coffees.

The antioxidants in coffee impart many health benefits, such as the following:

> Both decaffeinated and regular coffee turn off mTOR and switch on AMPK, which triggers autophagy [59]. Thus, coffee encourages the body to rejuvenate and repair the body's cells. We get the picture. We add a little coffee and exercise to our fasting regime and have three things kicking our bodies into autophagy.

> Regular coffee drinking reduces the risks of heart disease, Type II diabetes, and cancers such as liver, colorectal, and melanoma [249, 250].

> Coffee drinkers experience a lower risk of Alzheimer's, Parkinson's, and multiple sclerosis [249].

Coffee, or the caffeine in coffee, acts as a mild diuretic, causing the coffee drinker to urinate frequently. Fasters should drink beverages with no caffeine to replenish the body's water.

Bulletproof coffee has become popular with fasters. Nevertheless, there may be better choices than bulletproof coffee for intermittent fasting with fasting periods of less than 24 hours because the faster essentially drinks a liquid meal.

Bulletproof coffee clocks in the calories. The typical recipe is one cup of brewed coffee blended with two tablespoons of unsalted butter, two tablespoons of coconut oil (medium chain triglycerides), and two tablespoons of heavy cream. Thus, the coffee has nearly six tablespoons of fat and packs 648 calories. The calorie count depends on the recipe and which ingredients the person blends with the coffee. Some fasters substitute a strong tea for coffee to make bulletproof tea.

We can estimate the calorie content of bullet coffee or tea. One teaspoon of fat equals 4 grams. A tablespoon equals three teaspoons and thus 12 grams of fat. A gram of fat holds 9 calories of energy. Hence, one tablespoon of fat yields 108 calories. We can ignore the calories in the coffee or tea since it adds four or fewer calories than the fat.

A person fasting beyond 24 hours or following the ketogenic diet may benefit from drinking bulletproof coffee. The coffee should keep the person in a state of ketosis, but the person burns fat from the coffee and not the fat stored in his or her body.

I have tried bulletproof coffee. It tastes similar to a rich cup of cappuccino since the blender froths the cream. However, we are drinking a liquid meal.

Exogenous Ketones

We constantly search for ways to strengthen the state of ketosis without having to fast beyond two days. Unfortunately, the body quickly adapts to fasting. In one study, healthy women experienced a drop in a blood ketone, beta-hydroxybutyrate, during their second fast [251]. This study presents trouble because ketones may signal cells to switch on autophagy and the longevity genes, sirtuins [65]. Furthermore, ketones may rejuvenate senescent cells and activate the stem cells when the feasting cycle starts again. Then the liver can create glucose from both proteins and glycerol because the body's cells prefer sugar as its primary energy source. Thus, the body does its best to overcome the stress of fasting.

Exogenous ketones, which are salts of beta-hydroxybutyrate, could help strengthen the state of ketosis. The salts also supply the body with minerals such as calcium, magnesium, and sodium, which leads to our next tip.

> ➤ **Tip #29:** In theory, a faster can take exogenous ketones to strengthen the state of ketosis since many of the health benefits of fasting are associated with the level of beta-hydroxybutyrate in the blood. Sometimes, we take exogenous ketones around 20 hours into a 24-hour or longer fast.

When I returned to the United States, I bought exogenous ketones at Walmart. I experimented and took 345 mg of exogenous ketones 20 hours into a 30-hour fast. An intense fasting euphoria swept through my mind and lasted for the remainder of the fast. I usually fast beyond 30 hours to get that incredible fasting euphoria. In addition, I do not take the exogenous ketones at the beginning of a fast because my body is burning the excess glucose from my diet. The 20 hours of fasting help the body burn the excess sugar because the body's cells prefer glucose first before consuming ketones for energy. It is possible to induce ketoacidosis if taking exogenous ketones simultaneously with a high carbohydrate diet [16]. High levels of both fuels turn the blood acidic, which is dangerous.

Some people rate exogenous ketones poorly because they have overloaded their diet with carbohydrates. Subsequently, exogenous ketones have little impact on their bodies since most cells consume glucose first as their primary fuel before consuming fats and ketones.

Flavored Water

Fasters can drink flavored water. The faster squeezes fresh juice from either lemons or limes into water. One lemon contains about 24 calories, while one lime contains around 20 calories. Both include Vitamin C with the minerals – calcium, magnesium, phosphorus, and potassium. Many purport the health benefits of consuming fresh lemon or lime juice daily.

Fasters can use other fruits and vegetables to make flavored water. We can submerge berries, cucumber slices, or orange slices in water to infuse the water with flavor. Cucumbers are a good choice since they contain minuscule traces of sugar, while berries and oranges contain sugar. The sugar could kick the faster out of ketosis. Thus, we should be careful about which fruits we add when making flavored water.

The food industry offers vitamin and fiber water. Depending on the brand, we should avoid these. Many brands contain as much sugar as sodas and juices. Again, the sugar would throw the faster out of ketosis. Furthermore, the food industry offers zero-calorie vitamin and fiber waters, but they sweeten the water with artificial sugars or stevia. We do not know the long-term effects of artificial sugars on health and whether artificial sugars raise insulin levels in humans [252].

Soda Water

Although I am not enthusiastic about sugar sodas, I accidentally came across soda water. As an American, sometimes I should remember that some names do not translate well outside the United States. For example, I was visiting a friend in New Zealand and asked for a soda at a restaurant. Imagine the surprise when I sipped the water, which had no flavor or sweetness. It was just carbonated water. Duh! Soda is just carbonated water and not a carbonated sugary drink outside the United States. However, this accidental discovery changed my fasting life. I enjoy drinking soda water during a fast, which leads to our next tip.

> **Tip #30:** Soda water is refreshing and effervescent for people who love drinking their sugary carbonated drinks. It contains zero calories, and some companies add traces of minerals. Soda water is also called club soda, seltzer, and sparkling water.

Tea

Tea drinkers enjoy tea in a variety of flavors. We call tea a drink made from the plant's leaves, *Camellia Sinensis*. However, tea companies process the same leaf in many ways that change the taste, flavor, and cost of the tea. For example, tea companies mass produce teas cheaply using a special hedger that cuts the top leaves from the tea bush. Meanwhile, laborers handpick expensive, quality teas. The pickers remove the top three young leaves and buds of new growth.

Tea also differs in processing and includes the following:

> **White Tea:** Producers use young shoots from the tea bush and do not allow the tea to oxidize, making white tea the least processed tea [253]. Oxidation means that some chemicals in the

tea react with the oxygen in the air. Oxidation darkens the tea leaves and changes their flavors.

➢ **Green Tea:** Producers quickly dry the tea leaves to stop oxidation [253]. Green tea is slightly oxidized.

➢ **Oolong Tea:** Oolong tea lies between green and black and is partially oxidized [253].

➢ **Black Tea:** Producers completely oxidize the tea leaves, and it is the most commonly drunk tea in the Western world [253].

➢ **Matcha Tea:** Growers cover the tea bush for three weeks before harvest. Then producers pulverize the whole green tea leaf into a fine powder. Tea drinkers drink the entire leaf.

Fasters can enjoy tea during fasts without worry as long as they add no sugar or dairy products. Tea has zero or close to zero calories and trace minerals and vitamins [248]. Tea contains traces of calcium, magnesium, phosphorus, potassium, sodium, and zinc [248], but the nutrients depend on tea type, variety, and growing conditions.

It is possible to write another book on the health benefits of tea in all its varieties and forms. For instance, all tea from the *Camellia Sinensis* contain polyphenols, which are catechins, flavonoids, and theaflavins. These substances are antioxidants that have many health benefits. Antioxidants neutralize free radicals in the body. Free radicals are charged molecules floating around the body, harming and damaging cells and tissues; cigarette smoke, radiation, and the cells making energy create free radicals.

➢ **Tip #31 – Sun-Brewed Tea:** Place between 4 and 8 tea bags in a clear glass pitcher of water. Cover the pitcher to keep bugs out and expose it to at least four hours of direct sunlight. Sun-brewed tea has a milder taste than brewed tea and works well for inexpensive, bitter black teas. Then we drink it as an iced tea.

Fasters and health-conscious people focus on green tea because catechins suppress appetite, boost metabolism, and help lose weight [11]. Green tea also contains epigallocatechin gallate (EGCG) that triggers autophagy, or at least in the livers of mice [67]. Steeping tea leaves in hot water dissolve some of the antioxidants.

Matcha tea is another good choice. It started in Japan, where the Japanese pulverize the green tea leaf into a fine powder. That way, the tea drinker consumes all the nutrients and antioxidants from the tea leaf. All popular coffee shops make a matcha smoothie. Matcha tea contains up to 25 calories per cup because the producers add sugar. Sometimes, drinking matcha tea gives a little buzz, so the tea contains something. Matcha tea can be challenging to make, which is the next tip.

> ➢ **Tip #32** – Matcha Tea: The tea mixes poorly with water. The tea drinker places the matcha tea in a cup and adds a little hot water. Then the person uses a flat, small spoon to thoroughly dissolve the powder into the water before filling the cup with hot water. The tea clumps if not completely dissolved. Another method is to place the matcha tea in a capsule for espresso machines like Nescafe Dulce Gusto and Keurig. The machine works by dissolving the tea powder into the water using hot water and pressure.

Herbal tea excludes tea from the *Camellia Sinensis* and includes a mixture of herbs such as chamomile, jasmine, ginger, dried fruit, mint, lavender, hibiscus, or licorice. Many of these herbs impart health benefits in and of themselves, and many are also blended with tea from *Camellia Sinensis*. Of course, black tea with strawberry or tropical flavors is excellent, but fasters have many choices.

Tea is also a great drink when sick, which leads to the next tip.

> ➢ **Tip #33** – Ginger Tea: Clean and thinly slice a fresh ginger root. Place five slices of ginger in a black tea bag and steep in a cup of hot water. I learned this trick in Malaysia when I suffered from a persistent sore throat because ginger has antifungal, antibacterial, and antiviral properties. After two

days of drinking this tea twice daily, good riddance to the sore throat.

Vitamins and Minerals

Calcium, magnesium, phosphorus, and potassium levels stay remarkably stable in the body during a fast [17] along with proteins and vitamins [9]. However, the zinc levels rise in the blood, which results from the body catabolizing and breaking down tissues within the body [17]. In addition, the body loses sodium rapidly during a fast [17, 21, 31], which explains why the body sheds excess water with rapid weight loss [17, 21].

Some fasters take multivitamins and mineral supplements during their fast. However, Dr. Joel Fuhrman believes that one should avoid vitamin and mineral supplements during a fast to allow the complete rest of the digestive system [9]. Salt, i.e., sodium chloride, should be the only exception. Some fasters believe salt would violate their fast, while others do not. When my fast extends beyond 24 hours, I add a ½ teaspoon of Himalayan salt to my hot water, drink bone broth, or drop a bouillon cube into hot water.

We all heard the dangers of high salt and fats in our diets. The loss of salt during a fast shows that we fasters should not restrict our diets during our feasting cycles. Diet restriction could compound mineral and vitamin deficiencies over time. For example, we fast and lose some sodium. Then we feast but limit our salt intake. As we continue to fast and feast over months, we continually lose sodium until the sodium deficiency endangers our health. Furthermore, we should not restrict our oil and fat intake because these oils help our digestive system absorb vitamins A, D, E, and K. (Remember to eat your bananas because raising salt intake may lead to potassium loss).

We should take vitamins and minerals during our feasting cycles to ensure we have plenty of nutrients. One of my favorite supplements is Spirulina, a blue-green alga that grows in salty water in oceans and salty lakes in subtropical climates. Several celebrities call Spirulina the superfood because it contains significant amounts of amino acids, calcium, iron, magnesium, potassium, magnesium, and B vitamins [254]. Amino acids are the building blocks of proteins [254]. Proponents claim that Spirulina cures a variety of health conditions because it also contains beta-carotene (related to Vitamin A), phycocyanin (blue pigment), and tocopherols (related to Vitamin E) [254]. However, I do not offer any health claims for Spirulina. I take Spirulina because I call it God's natural multivitamin. It comes from nature.

Yeast extract, an alternative to Spirulina, contains vitamin Bs, minerals, and protein. Yeast, a fungus, decomposes sugar into ethanol and carbon dioxide and forms the backbone of the beer and wine industry. Furthermore, yeast undergoes autolysis, where the yeast cells break down into simpler components, which we call yeast extract when the yeast dies.

Yeast extract contains proteins called glutamates. The food industry uses monosodium glutamate (MSG) as a flavor enhancer and extracts MSG from the yeast extract. Some blame MSG for headaches, allergies, and infant obesity. The food industry uses MSG and yeast extract interchangeably. We usually find MSG in bouillon cubes. Thus, I occasionally enjoy a bouillon cube in a mug of hot water during a fast.

We should do our research to determine which supplements are best for us. Supplements are expensive, and people should avoid taking a whole assortment of them. Other supplements for anti-aging include acetyl-L-carnitine arginate, CoQ10, green tea extract, pycnogenol (French pine bark), and resveratrol (from grape skins). Just be careful. In rare cases, people taking green tea extract suffer from liver and kidney issues. That leads to the next tip.

> **Tip #34:** We should take vitamin and mineral supplements on our feasting days to ensure our bodies have plenty of nutrients for our fasting days. My favorites include fish oil, vitamin B3, and Spirulina.

The health food industry creates vitamin and mineral supplements from chemical processes. Some people debate whether the human body can utilize artificial chemicals. For example, beta-carotene, a precursor to Vitamin A, imparts many health benefits to the human body. However, beta-carotene in pill forms does not provide the same benefits as natural beta-carotene from carrots and orange vegetables. If given a choice, we should always choose natural sources to sustain our nutritional needs.

Vaping and Smoking

A section on vaping and smoking is included because several young people ask whether smoking cigarettes or vaping breaks a fast. Technically, a person does not eat tobacco, so the digestive system does not process the chemicals in tobacco. It also does not appear to spike insulin. Therefore, the tobacco does not break a fast. However, consuming tobacco products breaks the "spirit" of the fast because a person fasts to remove the toxins and poisons from the body. Consuming a tobacco product introduces new toxins and poisons into the body during a fast. For instance, the primary chemical, nicotine, stimulates the body at low dosages but turns into a poison at high dosages. In addition, cigarette smoke contains about 4,000 toxins, which create free radicals in the body [63]. Then the free radicals damage cells. It is important to note that while smoking and vaping do not technically break a fast, they do introduce toxins and poisons into the body, which may affect your overall health.

Two studies highlight the dangers of nicotine. First, nicotine could lead to insulin resistance and hinder the action of insulin in the body for both smoking and nicotine gum [255]. (We can assume vaping would impart the same effect on the body). We already know that insulin allows the cells to utilize glucose for energy and encourages the body to store glucose as fat. Nevertheless, insulin resistance leads to metabolic syndrome – high blood pressure, diabetes, heart disease, and obesity. Second, the free radicals in second-hand smoke and cigarette smoke damage the mitochondria in the cells [63]. The mitochondria are the energy furnaces inside the cells. Although this is another study of mice, the damaged mitochondria switch on autophagy as the cells break down the damaged mitochondria and produce new ones [63]. Thus, we have a dilemma. If a person did not smoke that cigarette, his or her body could be repairing other cells instead of the recently damaged cells from the cigarette smoke. Remember, in Chapter 3, we discussed the epigenetic theory of aging. Sirtuins must go and fix the DNA or repair the mitochondria. If the sirtuins do not return, the cell ages because it cannot unravel the DNA from the histones to read it. Thus, the cells age at the cellular level.

Do not get me wrong. I am not an anti-smoking crusader. Sometimes, I enjoy a cigar while drinking with friends. I also vaped when it was cool in 2014. The key is moderation; I enjoy about four cigars yearly, but not every day. The emphasis is on moderation, and it empowers us to make informed choices about our health and wellness.

7. Fasting Diets

"When the stomach is full, it is easy to talk of fasting."
– St. Jerome

The key to fasting is sustainability and attitude. We fast regularly to cleanse and repair the body. We utilize an ancient system into our bodies and turned it into a bio-hack. The body, just like our house, needs periodic cleaning. Fasting also helps nullify most of the adverse effects of aging. However, a person's attitude determines whether that person will fast or not. For example, my best friend is a brilliant researcher and professor at a university in New Zealand. Unfortunately, he is encountering many health problems in his 40s – chronic infections, severe allergies, and digestion system problems, including sensitivity to wheat gluten. He sees how fasting has made me healthy but refuses to fast. Unfortunately, he was forced to fast as part of his religious duties as a child, and he detests fasting. This is quite common. People forced to do something turn them off from doing something voluntarily.

On the other hand, I look forward to a fast. I have two whole days a week where I do not prepare meals or wash dishes. I am also getting the health benefits outlined in this book. Thus, I enjoy my fasts with a good cup of coffee and a dash of heavy cream.

In this chapter, fasters can incorporate fasting into their lifestyle. Fasters must experiment to find which regimen works well for them. For example, some fast people swear by one meal a day (OMAD) and how this diet has transformed their lives. I love food, so I cannot do this fasting regimen. Instead, I fast between 24 and 36 hours and feast for two days. If I do a 48-hour fast, I feed for at least four days. Then I eat like a condemned man eating his last meal before his execution during feasting days.

This chapter not only provides ideas on how to incorporate fasting into your life but also highlights the relationship between fasting and other diets. It is important to note that fasting can complement other diets, such as the ketogenic and fasting-mimicking diets. The ketogenic diet, for instance, activates the same pathways as fasting [66], making it a potential partner in your fasting journey.

The Ketogenic Diet

Medical doctors started the ketogenic diet in the 1920s to treat children's epilepsy. The name ketogenic comes from the word ketone. The diet became popular in the 1920s and 1930s and has recently resurged in popularity. Celebrities go on the keto diet and show off their toned, chiseled bodies.

The ketogenic diet does not involve fasting since the dieter still eats food. Thus, the ketogenic diet is weaker than water fast because all food elicits an insulin response except pure fats [12]. Nobody eats pure fat. However, the Keto diet puts the dieter into a perpetual state of ketosis and resembles the process of fasting, when the body burns fat for energy. The dieter either burns fat from his or her body or the fat from the food. The diet produces ketones, i.e., beta-hydroxybutyrate, acetoacetate, and acetone. The ketones send the body's cells the starvation signal, which switches on some of the health benefits of fasting [16].

Some believe the ketogenic diet is not strong enough to reverse insulin resistance [11]. Some people need a fast to reset their insulin levels. Furthermore, some people combine the ketogenic diet and intermittent fasting to multiply the health benefits of both regimens.

The U.S. Departments of Agriculture and Health and Human Services recommend consuming between 20 and 35% fat, 10 and 35% protein, and the remaining calories from carbohydrates. The keto diet recommends around 70% of fat, 25% protein, and 5% carbohydrates. Women require 2,000 calories daily and would restrict their carbohydrates to 100 calories or lower for the keto diet. Meanwhile, on average, men consume 2,500 calories daily and would limit their carbs to 150 calories or lower. In practice, dieters often restrict carbs to 50 calories or lower.

The ketogenic diet restricts carbohydrates extremely. Table 5 shows how much carbs a dieter can eat in one day. Dieters are limited to a tiny fruit daily or a 1/3 cup of cooked brown rice. Starbucks lovers can have a caffe latte with nonfat milk or two cold brew coffees with almond milk, but other Starbucks drinks and cakes are forbidden. Once dieters consume their tiny carb portion, they are left with proteins and fat for the remainder of the day. In addition, the dieters must control their protein intake since the liver can manufacture glucose from protein.

We see that the keto diet is extreme regarding carbohydrate restriction. Some people experience the Keto flu as the body adapts to burning fat as energy. The symptoms resemble the flu and include diarrhea, dizziness, headache, nausea, vomiting, and weakness [256]. The symptoms can last a week [256]. Technically, the dieters experience sugar withdrawal symptoms as the dieter experiences extreme sugar cravings. Other Keto complications include the Keto crotch, where the crotch emits strong smells.

Table 5. Foods with Approximately 50 Calories in Carbs

Fresh Fruit	
One small apple with skin	One orange
One small banana	One small peach
Two slices pineapple	Watermelon, a cup, diced

Bread	
Three slices white bread	Six saltine crackers
One slice wheat bread	Ten wheat crackers

Starbucks	
One Caffe Latte with nonfat milk	
Two cold brewed coffees with almond milk	

Miscellaneous	
1/3 cup cooked brown rice	¼ cup white rice

Source: Calorie King [257]. The approximate amount is calculated by subtracting the fiber in grams from total carbohydrates. Then multiply by four to yield calories from carbs. The digestive system does not break down the fiber into sugar. Instead, it passes the fiber to the stool.

Many nutritionists and doctors debate the long-term health problems of a keto diet. In a mouse study, a high-fat diet raised LDL cholesterol and increased ratios of cholesterol/HDL and LDL/HDL [88]. Hence, the researchers are setting up the little critters for future heart attacks. In another study of rats, scientists show that the ketogenic diet switches off mTOR in liver and brain cells [52]. The mTOR pathway must be turned off to promote autophagy. Although we share similar biological processes with mice, research studies often do not transfer to humans.

In a human study, researchers studied the keto diet on 15 military personnel, with 14 people in the control group. The control group showed no change during the study. On the other hand, the keto group lost 16.9 pounds (or 7.7 kg), lost visceral fat, and experienced an improvement in insulin sensitivity [258]. The study lasted 12 weeks, and both groups ate until they were satisfied [258]. The keto group showed the same athletic performance as the control group in squats, bench presses, sprints, and other exercises [258]. The study confirmed that the keto group entered ketosis after three days [258]. Although they are not fasting, we see the three days again. Finally, the study has one flaw – the participants chose which group to join [258]. Thus, we have a selection bias with the keto group. Perhaps the keto group was chubbier and wanted to diet.

In another human study, the cholesterol, LDL, and HDL levels were similar on high-fat and low-fat diets [259]. The high-fat diet comprised 39% of fat, while the low-fat diet comprised 22%. The high-fat diet is not the ketogenic diet. However, the subjects on a low-fat diet exhibited higher triglyceride levels [259], indicating their bodies converted the excess sugar into triglycerides.

We must remember that table sugar is half glucose and half fructose. The liver manufactures triglycerides from excess fructose in the body. Dr. George Bray believes a diet high in fructose increases triglycerides because the liver turns fructose into fat [260]. That is why we should avoid sodas and drinks brimming with high-fructose corn syrup.

News reporters, of course, love reporting sensational news that the keto diet will harm the dieters and their health. We must be careful when we cite and read research papers. That is why I added the mouse study. Perhaps researchers saw an increase in cholesterol in mice. Let us say they stopped the study and dissected the mice before they developed heart disease. Then in the conclusion, they cite a paper that connects high cholesterol levels to heart disease in mice. Bam, high-fat diets cause heart disease in mice. The news reporters get a hold of this research paper and write a news story about how the ketogenic diet leads to heart disease in humans.

Research is not dishonest per se. We play a game because research is like hitting a home run. We will triumph if we get our article published in a top-notch journal. Our employers and the universities love us and shower their top researchers with promotions, reduced teaching hours, and other benefits. If our employer does not respect us, the top researchers can relocate to another university. Unfortunately, professors who are excellent teachers but poor researchers may have trouble finding new employment opportunities.

The research presents another problem. The research literature contains several conflicting studies. We can easily find another research study on mice that shows a high-fat diet does not affect cholesterol. This is not dishonest. Perhaps one group of researchers used mice prone to high cholesterol levels, while the second group did not. When we write that brilliant research article, we emphasize research papers that support our ideas and de-emphasize papers that weaken our ideas. It does not matter if one person reads our research paper. We hit a home run. Then we show our employer and earn our rewards.

Grant money may complicate research and lead to biased research reports. Our employers expect us to go out and obtain research funding. They give it a cute name – monetizing research. Universities are just as hungry and greedy for money as corporations, but we posit altruistic reasons why we need the money. Therefore, when we receive a research grant, we must substantiate the claim the granter wants. Otherwise, that benefactor will never grant us a research grant again.

A large corporation, for example, bestows a multimillion grant to study the health effects of one of its products, high fructose corn syrup (HFCS). Some claim that HFCS causes fatty liver, insulin resistance, and high triglyceride levels [12, 260] and, in addition, increases the risk of obesity, diabetes, and heart disease [260]. Researchers must find ways to amplify the positive benefits of HFCS and de-emphasize its negative qualities. Otherwise, the corporation will never fund the researchers again. Thus, we must be careful when reading and citing research papers. This may be why numerous conflicting studies and reports dominate the research literature.

Unfortunately, we see problems with the keto diet. The U.S. Department and the food industry have demonized fats since the 1970s. The food industry offers a large variety of high-carb, low-fat snacks. The keto diet has come along and threatens to shake up the food industry. Then we read and listen to the many conflicting research news on how the keto diet ruins (improves) our health and quickens (slows) our destination to our final resting spot.

Sometimes, I may eat one or two meals that are extremely low in carbohydrates and high in fats before starting a fast. I can tell it strengthens the fast. Consequently, we can go on the ketogenic diet one or two days before the start of the fast, which leads to the next tip.

> ➤ **Tip #35:** Fasters can go on the ketogenic diet before starting a fast. The keto diet puts the person into ketosis before the fast, strengthening short-term fasts. Dieters can break a fast with a keto meal to extend their state of ketosis.

Because of the keto diet, I boosted the fats in my diet. However, the diet has a large impact on training. For example, I love carbohydrates and usually train on a high-carb diet. One time, I ate several low-carbohydrate meals a day before a 10-kilometer run. I felt great. I experienced no pain. Once I reached the 7-kilometer mark, I lost all my energy and had to walk the remaining distance. The problem is I do not train on the ketogenic diet. I am used to the sugar fuel for the initial energy during a run. Consequently, athletes going on the ketogenic diet must train while on the diet to maintain their performance.

Keto Diet Health Benefits

Are we surprised that the ketogenic diet offers health benefits? The keto diet restricts carbohydrates that our bodies break down into glucose. Then the liver starts making a substitute fuel - beta-hydroxybutyrate for our bodies.

One study surveyed 135,335 people in 18 countries. We must be careful of these studies because the researchers ask participants to complete surveys [261]. The researchers found that the group who ate the highest quantity of carbohydrates had the highest incidence of mortality [261]. This group also suffered from the highest incidence of myocardial infarctions, stroke, and cardiovascular disease [261]. The group who ate the most saturated or unsaturated fats had the lowest incidence of strokes [261].

The ketogenic diet raises the level of ketones circulating in the bloodstream. The mitochondria burn ketones more efficiently than glucose, which raises NAD+ [262]. We already read that the longevity genes, sirtuins, rely on NAD+ to produce their enzymes. Consequently, ketones may activate SIRT1 and SIRT3 [16], the same ones that fasting activates. The sirtuins are involved in lowering inflammation, helping the mitochondria burn energy more efficiently, and repairing DNA. Ketones may also activate AMPK, which switches on autophagy [16].

The ketogenic diet reduces insulin levels [16]. We have already learned that high insulin levels may cause inflammation and insulin resistance. Beta-hydroxybutyrate also reduces inflammation directly [263] and may improve heart health because the heart relies on ketones for energy [16]. Consequently, the ketogenic diet boosts the heart's primary fuel source.

The ketogenic diet may be effective against some forms of cancer. In one experiment, mice had glioma, a cancer cell that forms tumors in the brain and spinal cord. The glioma forms from glial cells, which are cells that support the neurons. A glioma is particularly nasty since it can spawn cancerous stem cells [264], which means it can mutate into different cancerous cells. Gliomas are challenging to treat because of their stem cell nature, and they depend on sugar (i.e., the Warburg effect) for energy [264]. Switching the body's metabolism to ketosis causes these cancerous cells to starve and die since they cannot utilize ketones for fuel [264]. The ketones damage the cancer cells' mitochondria and induce apoptosis in some cancer cells [264].

I started restricting my carb intake and did not follow the keto diet strictly. I shop at the grocery and health stores and buy a variety of delicious keto treats, snacks, and desserts. Thus, we can strategically utilize the ketogenic diet to strengthen the effects we get from fasting and manufacture those ketones in our bodies a little longer.

The Fasting-mimicking Diet

Valter Longo, the director of the University of Southern California Longevity Institute, created the fasting-mimicking diet [265]. The diet allows people to benefit from fasting without completely abstaining from food [266].

The diet lasts five days and uses the following protocol:

> On the first day, the dieter consumes 1,090 calories. The meals contain 56% fat, 34% carbohydrates, and 10% protein [266, 267].

> On the remaining days, the dieter eats 725 calories daily. The meals contain 44% fat, 47% carbohydrates, and 9% protein [266, 267].

Day 1 is a transition day, but interestingly, Day 1 has the highest calories from fat, while the remaining days have the highest calories from carbs. The carbohydrates would kick the faster out of the fasting state, but the diet makes up for the carbohydrates by fasting for five days. Researchers claim that the fasting-mimicking diet is ketogenic even though the carbohydrates appear too high [99]. However, the calories are limited, and the carbohydrates may not be high enough to kick the fasters out of the fasting state.

The company, L-Nutra, sells ProLon meal kits to help people implement the fasting-mimicking diet [265]. The meal kits sell between $250 and $300, depending on how many kits a consumer purchases [265]. Over 52,000 people have purchased meal kits [265]. That means the company has grossed at least $13 million. Not bad. Hence, one company found a way to make money from fasting.

People may find the diet helpful, but we require reliable postal service. I do not trust the Malaysian postal service to deliver an expensive package to my door. Sometimes, I receive my mail; sometimes, I don't. I remember it took the postal service four months to deliver an urgent bank letter.

> **Tip #36:** Some fasters require a crutch to help them transition to fasting. A meal kit comes in handy. The faster does not need to measure his or her food or count the grams of fat, carbohydrates, and proteins. Thus, the meal kit makes fasting easier and more convenient.

Professor Valter Longo conducts much-needed research into fasting using his fasting-mimicking diet. I read several of his team's papers, and their papers are good and published in top journals. However, the research indirectly benefits the L-Nutra company, which he founded. He donates 60% of his profits to Create Cures Foundation, a non-profit organization that applies science to the treatment of diseases. Professor Longo is also the founder. The good news is that his research team studies fasting at the cellular level.

In one study, for example, researchers showed that mice on a fasting-mimicking diet experienced a boost in the number of stem and progenitor cells upon refeeding [266]. Stem cells are blank cells that the body uses to repair damaged cells in tissues and organs. Progenitor cells are similar to stem cells, except they are more limited in which cells they transform into.

In mice studies, researchers found that a two-day or three-day fast-mimicking diet cleans and clears the blood of senescent white blood cells [100, 239]. Then the immune system quickly regenerates white blood cells upon refeeding [239]. Stem cell regeneration comes with a drawback. If a faster exposes him- or herself to carcinogenic substances during refeeding, he or she may transform those new cells into cancerous cells [37, 103].

Popular Fasting Diets

Several diets gained popularity. These are not actual diets where the dieter restricts his or her food choices. They use a combination of feeding and fasting windows. The diets are ranked from the easiest to the most difficult as the fasting window increases or the number of fasts per week increases.

- ➢ **LeanGains or 16:8:** Marin Berkhan popularized this regimen, in which the dieter eats all his daily food during an eight-hour window and fasts for the remaining 16 hours [268]. Dieters maintain flexibility and determine their eating window, such as joining the family for supper. The 18:6 regimen is also popular, with a six-hour eating window and an 18-hour fast.

- ➢ **Eat Stop Eat or 5:2:** A person fasts for two days out of the week and freely eats during the remaining five days [10, 268]. Michael Mosley, a British journalist, popularized a version of the diet by allowing the dieter to eat up to 500 calories daily for a woman and 600 calories for a man on a fasting day [10]. The dieter spreads the calories over the day or consumes all in one meal.

- ➢ **The Warrior Diet or 20:4:** A faster eats all his daily meals within a four-hour window and fasts for the remaining 20 hours [268]. Ori Hofmekler based his regimen on the eating habits of warriors who battled during the day and returned to the camp at night to feast [268].

- ➢ **Alternate-Day Fasting:** Dr. James Johnson popularized this eating protocol, in which a person fasts for a whole day and then feasts the next day [268]. Then the faster repeats.

- ➢ **The Snake Diet:** A person eats like a snake. The snake gulps down a rodent and lets its digestive system devour the rodent over a day or week. Thus, a person eats all meals within a one- or two-hour feeding window and fasts for the remaining time

[269]. Cole Robinson, the diet's creator, recommends the faster drink snake juice – a concoction of water and minerals [269].

> **One Meal a Day (OMAD):** The diet resembles the snake diet but omits the snake juice. The dieter eats all calories in a one-hour eating window and fasts for the remaining 23 hours of the day [270]. Blake Horton offers a diet similar to the OMAD [271]. He shocks the viewers on YouTube as Blake gorges on a mountain of food within an hour. He demonstrates the power of intermittent fasting.

> **The Autophagy Fast or Monk Fast:** The person eats regularly on his or her feasting day until 6 PM. On the second day, the person fasts for the whole day. Then the person resumes eating breakfast at 6 AM on the third day, granting the faster a 36-hour fast. Of course, we may adjust the time to conform to our schedules.

> **The Weekly Super Cleanse:** A person drinks only water for a fast between 42 and 60 hours once per week. I developed this fast because I regularly fast for at least 24 hours twice weekly. Instead of spacing out the two fasts, I joined them together. That way, a 48-hour fast imparts more benefits than a 24-hour fast because a person stays in autophagy longer. The digestion system processes and clears the food out once during a 48-hour fast rather than clearing the digestive system twice for two 24-hour fasts. Furthermore, the feasting and fasting days maintain a ratio of two to one, so people eat well during their feasting cycle for four days to prevent nutritional deficiencies.

The Autophagy Fast and Weekly Super Cleanse are the most beneficial. I am particularly interested in extending my life with minimum health problems, and these regimens have helped me achieve that. After all, what is the point of living forever if we are always sick and ill? That is why the ancient Greeks believed longevity and youth go together.

"To starve is to die; to fast is to live."

– Dr. Herbert Shelton

In this chapter, we explore the obesity epidemic in the United States, pinpointing its potential causes. There are many potential, interrelated causes. We then delve into the traditional methods employed by the healthcare industry to tackle obesity, including calorie restriction, exercise, and bariatric surgery.

The Obesity Epidemic

The obesity epidemic has exploded in the United States in the last fifty years. Obese people usually build layers of visceral fat around their organs in the abdomen. Visceral fat increases the risk of developing diabetes, hypertension, high cholesterol, hyperlipidemia (excess blood fat), liver problems, and heart disease [136, 272, 273]. Obese people could also suffer from gallbladder disease, osteoarthritis, gout, breathing problems, and sleep apnea [272] when a sleeper's breathing stops.

Some researchers blame obesity for health problems, while others suggest obesity is a symptom. For example, one theory states that obesity leads to chronic inflammation because many fatty deposits send out hormones and chemical proteins called cytokines, allowing cells to communicate [128, 129]. Cytokines could cause chronic inflammation as they continually send messages to the immune system. Then the immune system starts attacking healthy cells and tissues. Many of the diseases and illnesses in Chapter 2 originate from chronic inflammation.

How do we define obesity? Healthcare providers define obesity using the body mass index (BMI). The BMI equals a person's weight in kilograms divided by the person's height in squared meters [12, 274]. For example, before I discovered fasting, I weighed 220 pounds (or 100 kg) with a height of 5 ft 9 in (or 1.75 m). As calculated in Equation (1), my BMI equaled 32.7. Therefore, I was obese. This simple measure estimates I was 32.7% of fat. After six months of intermittent fasting, my BMI dropped to 28.4. Hurray, I am overweight.

$$BMI = \frac{weight\ in\ kilograms}{height\ in\ meters^2} = \frac{100}{1.75^2} = 32.7 \qquad (1)$$

The formula in (2) converts the measurements to a height in inches and weight in pounds.

$$BMI = 704.5 \times \frac{weight\ in\ pounds}{height\ in\ inches^2} = 704.5 \times \frac{220}{69^2} = 32.5 \quad (2)$$

The health professionals and doctors use Table 6 to classify their patients' BMI. The BMI assumes a person with a specific height carries a healthy body weight. A person with a BMI exceeding 35 has a 100-fold increase in the risk of diabetes [136]. Nevertheless, the BMI is not always accurate. The BMI incorrectly identifies bodybuilders and muscular men and women as overweight or obese even though they have a lean body mass.

Table 6. Body Mass Index (BMI) Classification

BMI Range	Classification
Less than 18.5	Underweight
18.5 – 24.9	Normal weight
25.0 – 29.9	Overweight
30.0 – 39.9	Obese
Greater than 40.0	Severely Obese

Source: National Center for Health Statistics [275]

We use the BMI to estimate obesity in the United States, as shown in Figure 2. The graph defines the percentage of Americans age 20 and older who are overweight, obese, or severely obese. The percentage removes the effect of a growing U.S. population. Ironically, the proportion of overweight people has remained constant since the 1960s. Only a few writers and researchers comment on this. However, obesity and severe obesity have skyrocketed over the same time.

Figure 2. U.S. Overweight and Obesity Trends, 2016

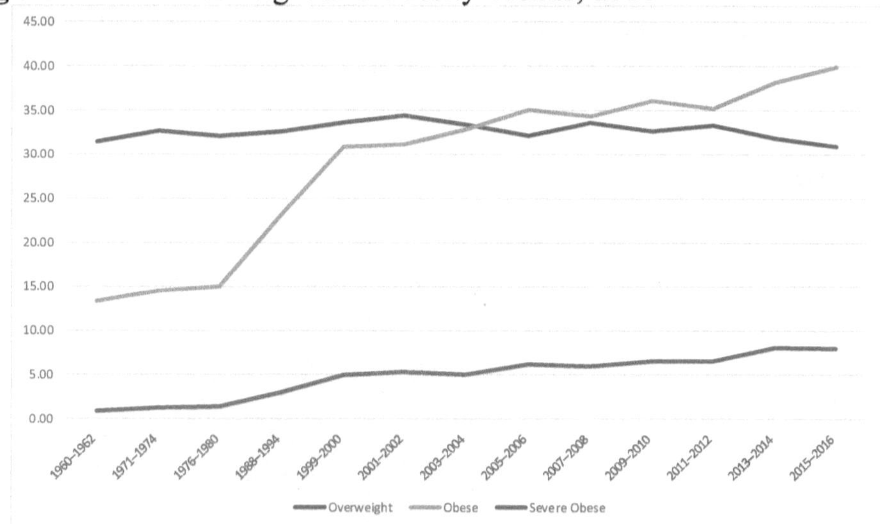

Source: National Center for Health Statistics [275]

Obesity does not strike all states, ethnic groups, and educational levels equally. The map in Figure 3 shows that California and Colorado have the lowest incidence of obesity, while the Southern United States has the highest. Usually, obesity strikes the poorest people, while educated people exhibit lower levels of obesity. Obesity also differs by ethnic group.

Scientists and doctors do not know why obesity is exploding so rapidly worldwide. The United States is the obesity capital of the world, while the United Kingdom is the obesity capital of Europe. Meanwhile, I reside in Malaysia, which has become the obesity capital of Asia.

The scientists and doctors posit several reasons to explain the explosion of obesity:

➤ The U.S. Department of Agriculture released its dietary guidelines in 1977 that encouraged a high-carbohydrate and low-fat diet [11, 12]. Many nations followed the United States such as the food labeling laws. The food labels in Malaysia resemble the United States. We have known for some time that

161

a diet high in carbohydrates makes people overweight. Two centuries ago, Jean Anthelme Brillat-Savarin (1755–1826) wrote that a diet high in flour and starch leads to obesity [276]. Remember, our digestive systems quickly break down flour and starches into glucose, i.e., sugar.

Figure 3. The Incidence of Obesity by State, 2016

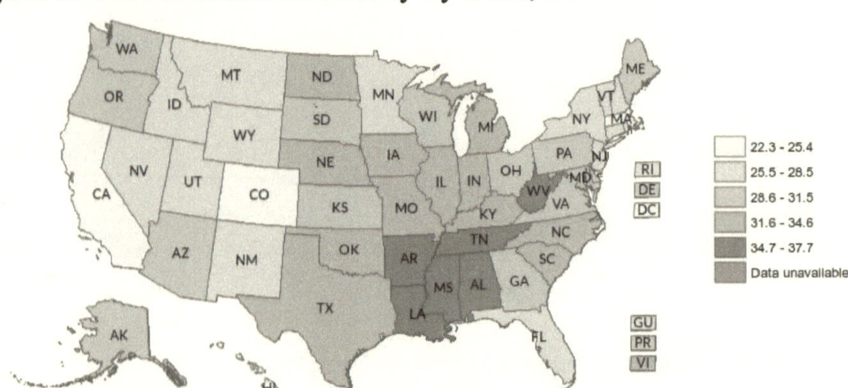

Source: Centers for Disease Control and Prevention [277]

Ironically, in 1972, a British medical doctor, Dr. John Yudkin, warned the public about high sugar consumption in his book *Pure, White, and Deadly*, explaining how it leads to diabetes and heart disease [278]. The public and medical field ignored his research and book for 30 years. However, Yudkin's book is witnessing a resurgence, and his words have turned into prophecy.

➢ The American society has witnessed the explosion of the snack food industry. Snack foods contain various types of sugar and refined carbohydrates. Even low-fat snacks make up the taste by adding sugar. In addition, the processing removes fiber, healthy vitamins, and minerals. Many U.S. snack foods are available everywhere in the world.

➢ Farmers have grown fruits and vegetables on the same land for decades. Some theorize that soils have become depleted in minerals. Thus, we eat more fruits and vegetables to compensate for the deficient nutrients [12].

➢ Families traditionally ate three meals: breakfasts, lunch, and dinner in 1977. By 2003, families snack between meals, so on average, a person eats up to six meals daily [11, 12]. The constant snacking leads to high insulin levels [12]. Then people become insulin resistant over time as they convert their bodies into sugar burners.

We assume modern families eat more calories from snacking because the evidence suggests meal frequency does not influence obesity [279, 280]. As long as a person eats the same calories, it makes no difference if that person snacks seven small meals throughout the day or gorges on two [279, 280]. (It would be interesting to compare gorging one meal daily versus snacking since the one daily meal would put a person into the fasting state).

➢ U.S. food manufacturers started manufacturing high fructose corn syrup (HFCS) in the 1960s, which we find in many products at the supermarket. Some claim that HFCS damages health and leads to fatty liver, insulin resistance, and elevated triglycerides [12, 260]. Only the liver metabolizes the fructose and converts it into fat [12, 260]. On the other hand, almost every cell in the body uses glucose for energy [12]. We rarely find HFCS outside the United States because the U.S. imposes high tariffs on imported sugar. The exception is soda because the United States exports sodas, with Coca-Cola and Pepsi available anywhere in the world. Non-U.S. food manufacturers use real table sugar because sugar is cheaper than HFCS. (Please note that table sugar is 50% glucose and 50% fructose; fruit also contains fiber, vitamins, and minerals.)

➢ When I grew up in the 1970s, we treated eating out as a luxury. We ate out occasionally. Currently, not only do families eat out more often, but they also eat more fast food [12]. Fast food contains more fat, sugar, and salt.

➤ Growing up in the 1970s, my friends and I always played outside. We constructed forts and tree houses, played baseball and basketball, and rode bicycles everywhere. In modern times, many children, teenagers, and young people stay indoors watching TV or playing games on the computer. Adults are more sedentary as they sit behind their desks somewhere in a cubicle maze, punching numbers into spreadsheets on a computer.

➤ The stress level in our society has risen several notches. Employment, relationships, and friendships have become temporary and fleeting. Stress constantly bombards us as we worry about being unemployed or our mate has run off with someone else. Our bodies release cortisol from physical and psychological stress. The constant stress and cortisol raise blood glucose and insulin and cause weight gain [11, 12].

➤ Some people sleep poorly. Sleep deprivation increases cortisol levels and, hence, people gain weight [12].

➤ A new theory links gut microbes to allergies, gastric cancer, inflammation, Type 2 diabetes, cardiovascular disease, and metabolic syndrome [281, 282]. Obese people could have a different composition of microbes in their gut, making their intestines more permeable [281]. Thus, food and bacteria can easily pass through the intestines and into the body, leading to chronic inflammation and metabolic syndrome [281].

Once we put on the weight, it becomes virtually impossible to take the weight off. In one study, researchers tracked 76,704 males and 99,791 females in the United Kingdom [274]. They concluded that an obese man has one chance out of 210 of attaining an average body weight [274]. Meanwhile, females fared better with a 1 out of 124 [274]. Unfortunately, the odds worsen for severely obese. A morbidly obese man has a 1 out of a 362 chance of achieving average weight, while a woman has a 1 out of 608 [274]. Thus, we have better odds of winning the jackpot in Las Vegas than losing weight. Finally, the study highlighted the problem of losing weight; at least half will regain the lost weight.

We are not sure why obesity is rising and what causes it. Once a person becomes obese, he or she will likely remain obese. Nobody wakes up in the morning and says I want to be obese. Trust me. I hit many hours in the gym and restricted my caloric intake, but I spent the last 30 years of my life being obese and trying to fight it. I did not conquer obesity until I started intermittent fasting. Wouldn't it be ironic that fasting regularly could solve the obesity epidemic and help people maintain a healthy weight?

Calorie-Restricted Diet

People practice calorie restriction when they purposely reduce their caloric intake. People watching their weight eat smaller portions and avoid sweets, pastries, and desserts. Calorie restriction imparts health benefits and helps reduce cancer [38, 99, 283]. Although not emphasized in this book, calorie restriction achieves many health benefits of fasting but has side effects. The constant restriction of food causes the dieters to become sensitive to cold, reduces their strength, and slows wound healing [99]. The calorie restriction could cause a loss of libido, infertility, and menstrual irregularities [99] because who wants to make love if they are cold and hungry? This hunger also makes the dieters more irritable, depressed, and obsessed with food [99], so they would not be pleasant to hang around.

Fasting resembles calorie restriction if fasting leads to lower food consumption. In a 12-week study, the experimental group reduced caloric intake by 300 calories daily during the 16:8 fasting regime [120]. Three hundred calories seem like little, but if this reduction is sustained over a year, it will be 31.3 pounds of fat yearly. However, they differ because fasting cycles the person between feasting and fasting. The fast also causes a rise in blood ketones that activate the stem cells and rejuvenate the senescent cells.

Fasting and calorie restriction could achieve identical weight loss [283], or the fasting group may experience greater weight loss [126]. However, fasters tend to lose less muscle than people on calorie-restricted diets [283].

Diet restriction causes other problems. We are limited on what we can restrict. We have three macronutrients: carbohydrates, proteins, and oils/fat. However, the number of diets we have is incredible. Nathan Pritikin started the first diet craze in America in 1979 with the publication of his bestseller - *Pritikin Program for Diet and Exercise*. The book advised dieters to eat a high-carbohydrate, high-fiber, and low-fat diet. The diet has one problem – the body burns sugar and carbohydrates quickly. Consequently, the dieter feels hungry again one or two hours after eating.

Then Dr. Adkin came along, advocated a high-protein diet, and started the next diet craze with Adkin's diet. The dieter eats copious amounts of protein and curtails carbohydrates [12]. Filling up with protein gives a person the feeling of satiety and fullness [12, 284].

Protein is one of those macronutrients we need because the body breaks it down into amino acids to build cells and tissues. We need about 0.36 grams per pound of body weight (or 0.8 grams per kg) [284]. That means I weigh 191.4 pounds (or 87 kg) and require a minimum of 68.9 grams of protein daily. On the other hand, bodybuilders and athletes need more protein to build and repair muscles.

Now, we are left with fats. The U.S. Department of Agriculture and the medical establishment demonize fats because fats pack twice the calories of proteins and carbohydrates. Each gram of fat provides 9 calories of energy, while carbohydrates and proteins supply 4 calories each. They also assume that the fat tissues in the body immediately absorb the fats from the diet. The establishment blamed fats for the increased body's cholesterol production, leading to heart disease and clogged arteries [12]. Like proteins, fats make the person feel full longer, which is why the ketogenic diet works.

The diets are further complicated because the macronutrients differ in quality. For example, an apple provides more nutrients than an apple pie. Fruits and vegetables lose vitamins and minerals from processing and cooking. Some health experts claim that vegetable oils like soybean, corn, and sunflower are inflammatory because they mainly comprise omega-6, six fatty acids [12]. Meanwhile, olive oil contains and balances omega three and omega six fatty acids and is considered healthier. Thus, olive oil is healthy for the heart [12]. Unfortunately, we are inundated with many diets and health tips.

Dr. Joel Fuhrman raises an excellent point about consuming high levels of animal proteins [9]. The fatty tissues of farm animals and fish concentrate pesticides, toxic chemicals, antibiotics, and growth hormones. Some doctors advise against high-protein diets and claim a high-protein diet leads to a large variety of diseases and health problems, such as cancer and atherosclerosis [9, 109]. The protein also flips the mTOR switch on and off autophagy [109]. Remember – autophagy allows cells to recycle protein from worn-out, damaged components in the cells. Thus, Dr. Fuhrman recommends that people obtain most of their proteins from fruits and vegetables [9].

One argument against the modern diet comes from Dr. Dewey, Dr. Shelton, and Mr. Sinclair. They noticed that many people suffered from health problems from consuming food at the turn of the 20th century [1-3]. People still become sick by eating a diet absent of all the chemicals, hormones, and toxins that exist in modern food. In addition, they only lived until 50 years old. Dr. Dewey noticed people were overeating and believed this overeating sparked many diseases [2].

Some claim that vitamin and mineral supplements in pill form are less effective than vitamins and minerals from plant sources. For example, fruits, vegetables, coffee, and tea contain phytochemicals, which act as antioxidants. Furthermore, some phytochemicals prevent cancer [9]. Therefore, Dr. Fuhrman recommends that people get their vitamins and minerals from plant sources [9].

All diets must ensure that every dieter gets his or her daily recommended vitamins and minerals. Deficiency in any vitamin or mineral causes health problems and diseases. Tables 7 and 8 show the minimum vitamins and mineral requirements for men and women aged between 31 and 50.

All diets suffer from the same problem: They restrict a person's food choices. For example, a person on a high-protein diet may crave carbohydrates such as ice cream and chocolate. A dieter on the Pritikin diet may tremble and shake for a hamburger with French fries. Thus, all diets are unsustainable and lead to a 99% failure rate [9, 11].

Table 7. Minimum Daily Vitamin Requirement

Vitamin	Chemical Name	Man	Woman
Biotin	Biotin	30 mcg	30 mcg
Choline	Choline	550 mg	425 mg
Vitamin A	Retinoids and carotene	900 mcg	700 mcg
Vitamin B1	Thiamin	1.2 mg	1.1 mg
Vitamin B2	Riboflavin	1.3 mg	1.1 mg
Vitamin B3	Niacin	16 mg	14 mg
Vitamin B5	Pantothenic Acid	5 mg	5 mg
Vitamin B6	Pyridoxine	1.3 mg	1.3 mg
Vitamin B9	Folic Acid	400 mcg	400 mcg
Vitamin B12	Cobalamin	2.4 mcg	2.4 mcg
Vitamin C	Ascorbic Acid	90 mg	75 mg
Vitamin D	Calciferol	15 mcg	15 mcg
Vitamin E	Alpha-Tocopherol	15 mg	15 mg
Vitamin K	Phylloquinone	120 mcg	90 mcg

Note: The table shows the minimum vitamin requirements for men and women between 31 and 50 years old. The acronyms stand for milligrams (mg) and micrograms (mcg).
Source: [285]

All diets have the following flaws:

➢ The degree of calorie restriction affects whether a person can follow a diet [286]. For example, a person who restricts daily calories by 10% is likelier to follow a diet than a person who restricts calories by 20%.

➢ Dieters lose weight initially, reach a plateau, and regain all the weight. They usually gain additional weight as a punishment [11, 12, 227].

Table 8. Minimum Daily Mineral Requirement

Mineral	Man	Woman
Calcium	1,000 mg	1,000 mg
Chloride	2.3 g	2.3 g
Chromium	35 mcg	35 mcg
Copper	900 mcg	900 mcg
Fluoride	4 mg	3 mg
Iodine	150 mcg	150 mcg
Iron	8 mg	8 mg
Magnesium	420 mg	320 mg
Manganese	2.3 mg	1.8 mg
Molybdenum	45 mcg	45 mcg
Phosphorus	700 mg	700 mg
Potassium	4.7 g	4.7 g
Selenium	55 mcg	55 mcg
Sodium	2,300 mg	2,300 mg
Sulfur	Unknown	Unknown
Zinc	11 mg	8 mg

Note: The table shows the minimum vitamin requirements for men and women between 31 and 50 years old. The acronyms stand for milligrams (mg) and micrograms (mcg).
Source: [285]

➤ Both the fasting and calorie-restricted groups lose weight. However, fasters experience greater weight loss in one study [126], identical weight loss in another [283], and less weight loss in another [136]. The calorie-restricted group showed no change in blood sugar level [136] or a decrease in blood sugar [126]. Meanwhile, the fasting groups showed declines in blood sugar [126, 136]. Ironically, the fasters and dieters showed increased insulin sensitivity [136], except in one study with overweight women [126]. The researchers believe that fasting women became less sensitive to insulin because the body reserves the scarce sugar for the brain and nervous system [126].

> Dieters experience a slowing metabolism [9, 11, 12, 273]. If a dieter restricts their consumption of calories by 10%, then that dieter's metabolism slows by 10% [12]. Furthermore, the diet restriction keeps the metabolism persistently slow [12, 227].

> Dieters feel miserable and hungry while their stomachs growl and grumble. Dieters become cold quickly and have trouble concentrating, while their blood pressure and heartbeat slow as the body conserves energy [12].

Diets fail because they always restrict people's choices for food. We want to eat the tasty, decadent, and rich food. How many people at the all-you-can-eat buffet reach for a steamed vegetable?

The famous TV show *The Biggest Loser* illustrates the problems of calorie-restricted diets and excessive exercise. The show pits two teams of dieters against each other to determine who loses the most weight. The last contestant wins and becomes the biggest loser.

The contestants exercised for several hours daily, eating healthy food in small portions. They lost an incredible amount of weight, with an average of 127 pounds (or 57.7 kg) of body weight [11], while their BMI dropped from 49% to 28% [11]. However, the weight loss was temporary! Kai Hibbard, who won the third season, said, "It was the biggest mistake of my life." In the second season, Suzanne Mendonca said, "There is never a reunion show because we're all fat again."

Researchers reviewed 14 contestants after six years after appearing on *The Biggest Loser* [227]. The contestants lost an average of 128.3 pounds (or 58.3 kg) and regained 90.2 pounds (or 41.0 kg) in six years [227]. Although the contestants lost some weight, their metabolism slowed to 704 calories daily [227]. That is a substantial decrease because a typical man requires about 2,500 calories, while a woman needs 2,000. Unfortunately, restricting calories slows down the metabolism.

That is why fasting works for some people. Intermittent fasting does not restrict food choices. It limits the feasting cycle for a brief time. Then fasters resume eating the foods they love and do not worry about their metabolism slowing down. We can also convert that decadent, high-calorie treat into an award, not a punishment.

Exercising

Many people exercise to lose weight. Exercise is classified as aerobic and anaerobic. Aerobic means "with oxygen," while anaerobic means "without oxygen." Both types build and strengthen the body.

People perform aerobic exercise when continually moving their bodies for a time. Running is the most intense aerobic exercise, but walking, swimming, cycling, or playing sports are also good for the body. Aerobic exercise strengthens the lungs, heart, and blood circulation because it places stress on the body. Consequently, the body becomes more efficient at transporting oxygen to the cells as the body burns energy to keep the constant motion.

Anaerobic exercise, on the other hand, involves short bursts of energy, the most common form being resistance training or weight lifting. The burst of energy causes the muscles to produce lactic acid from glucose. The buildup of lactic acid in the muscles gives the exerciser the feeling of burn or fatigue. Anaerobic exercise helps people develop speed, power, and strength, while bodybuilders pack on the bulging muscles on their frames.

Medical doctors always advise their patients to exercise to lose weight. However, exercise itself causes little weight loss. For example, I run on an elliptical trainer and burn 500 calories for 45 minutes twice per week. I also lift weights twice a week. At most, I burn 150 calories for a 30-minute workout.

I burned 52,000 calories in a year from running and 15,600 calories from weight lifting. I should lose 14.9 pounds (6.8 kg) from running and 4.5 pounds (or 2.0 kg) from weight lifting in one year. In 2017, my weight stayed at 220 pounds (or 100 kg) for the whole year. I lost no weight even though I exercised regularly during the year. A study confirms that exercise provides little weight loss. A study had three groups of women: A diet only, a diet with endurance exercise, and a diet with resistance exercise. All groups exhibited identical weight losses [286].

The body is an efficient, highly regulated machine. For instance, my body maintained my weight, although I was obese in 2017. What happened in 2017? I ate more to satisfy my hunger. Thus, I lost no weight. Furthermore, my hormones were out of balance, and the stress of the exercise could not correct the imbalance. The exercise also creates another effect. If we exercise in the gym for an hour, we reduce physical movement for other daily activities. For example, if I run for 45 minutes on the elliptical trainer, I stay home and watch a movie instead of strolling around in the mall.

I am not providing a reason for people to avoid exercise. Aerobic and anaerobic exercises impart many health benefits to the body. For example, running for 30 minutes switches the body from burning carbohydrates to burning fat for fuel. Frequent running imparts some of the health benefits of fasting. In addition, anaerobic exercise keeps muscles and bones strong. Strong, healthy muscles also burn more energy than the equivalent weight of fat. A good tip is combining an aerobic and anaerobic exercise regimen for optimal health.

> **Tip #37:** An excellent exercise program incorporates aerobic and anaerobic exercises.

Vanity comes with exercise. Being single in today's society is a challenge. It is not just the United States. The relationship crisis has hit many men and women around the world. I had women tell me that they could not find a good man. Then men say the same about finding a good woman. Thus, we have a severe mismatch problem as people stay single. Subsequently, many countries expect a declining population due to low birth rates.

Being athletic is a plus in today's society. I am not resurrecting the cavemen hypothesis that athletic men are more adept at catching prey to feed their women and children, while obese guys are dinosaur bait.

We, humans, desire something that we cannot have. It is similar to the diamond-water paradox that economists argued about in the 19th century. Diamonds are expensive and not essential for life. Meanwhile, water is cheap and essential for life. Hence, the paradox.

Of course, economists provide a simple answer. Water is abundant, while diamonds are scarce. An equal demand for both diamonds and water causes the market price for diamonds to exceed water greatly.

That is the same in dating. I live in Malaysia, the capital of obesity in Asia. Most people are chubby and want a skinny, athletic person for a mate. In the Middle Ages, most people were poor, malnourished serfs. Everybody was a chubby chaser because chubby males meant they ate and lived well, while chubby females indicated that the women would bear strong, healthy children. Thus, people are attracted to something rare, which today's modern society defines as skinny, athletic people living in a world drowning in plenty of cheap food.

Exercise programs are easy to start. We must invest in a good pair of sneakers, dress appropriately, and drink plenty of fluids for aerobic exercise. We can walk around the block for 30 minutes, toss a Frisbee with some friends, or play basketball or baseball with the kids. Some tips for starting an exercise regimen:

> **Tip #38:** We should consult a physician before beginning an exercise program if we are taking medications or suffering from a medical condition.

> **Tip #39:** We gradually ease into an exercise program. We do not run 10 kilometers on the first attempt. We start walking for 20 minutes and build strength and endurance over time.

> **Tip #40:** We must work out consistently at least two or three times per week. Exercising becomes easier over time. Unfortunately, we lose most of the aerobic benefits of exercise in as little as a month of no exercise.

> **Tip #41:** We exercise with a buddy to overcome boredom.

> **Tip #42:** We drink plenty of fluids to stay hydrated.

> **Tip #43:** We exercise outside because the sun and fresh air are also beneficial to the body.

➢ **Tip #44:** We do not exercise outside at noon when the summer sun scorches everything. During the summer, we exercise outside at dawn or dusk when the temperatures are cooler.

Many communities offer charity runs ranging between 3.1 miles (or 5 km) and a full marathon (26.2 miles or 42.2 km). These runs work well for people with a competitive nature. For example, I am extremely competitive. I sign up for a charity run every two months, usually between 3.1 miles (or 5 km) and 7.5 miles (or 12 km).

The charity run provides several benefits: First, the run motivates me to work out in the gym regularly. I want to ensure I am ready for the race. Second, I feed off the camaraderie and energy from the crowd of young, healthy people. I also love the stunned look my students give me as I pass by them during a race. Haha, uncle smoked them. Lastly, the races start early, around 6 AM, and the Island of Borneo has fantastic, vibrant sunrises. Then the runner's high kicks in while the sun rises.

Everybody gets a medal after crossing the finish line.

I proudly display my runner's bib and medal on my office wall. The runner's bib is the sweat-resistant number that a runner pins to his or her shirt.

People should complement aerobic exercise with resistance training to strengthen muscles and bones. Some tips when starting a weight training regimen include:

➢ **Tip #45:** Start a specific exercise with two repetitions with light weights. Over time, increase to at least three repetitions with heavier weights.

➢ **Tip #46:** People should warm up their muscles by running in place for five minutes or something similar.

➢ **Tip #47:** People should start working the largest muscles. The leg muscles are the largest in the body. The horizontal seat leg press hits the whole leg, including the calves, quads, glutes, and hamstrings. For more intense workouts, people can work up to barbell squats.

When we work out, we must remember to work symmetric opposing muscles. For example, the chest is the second largest group of muscles, and the symmetric opposing muscles are the back muscles.

> **Tip #48:** The chest and barbell bench press work the chest, biceps, and triceps. Then the lateral pull-down works on the large back muscles called the latissimus dorsi. Strengthening the latissimus dorsi gives athletes a triangular athletic look.

Other excellent exercises include:

1. Barbell shrugs exercise the trapezius, the top muscles that connect the shoulders to the neck. A person holds a heavy barbell in each hand and shrugs upward to exercise the trapezius.

2. The dip is a more advanced exercise that exercises the chest, front shoulders, and triceps. A person holds his body weight by grabbing onto the bars with both hands. Then the person plunges down and up vertically, similar to a vertical pushup. (Pull-ups work the opposite muscles of the dip.)

3. The shoulder press works the shoulders, trapezius, and triceps. A person sits in the machine and pushes the bar upward with his or her hands.

4. The bicep curl works the bicep muscles. A person holds a dumbbell in each hand and curls the barbell inward to work the muscle. We need the bicep curl to balance the tricep exercises in exercises (2) and (3) because the biceps and triceps are opposing muscles.

5. Leg raises or sit-ups work the abdominal muscles. Of course, we should not neglect the lower back muscles.

People should switch machines or techniques every few months to work the muscles differently. For example, the inclined or butterfly press works different parts of the chest muscles than the chest press. That way, the person exercises different muscles over time. We also talked about hormesis, where we constantly change our fasting regime to keep putting the body under different stresses.

We also have a choice in how we work out. If we are going to build muscle so that we can take on the Incredible Hulk, we should exercise with low repetitions and heavy weights. If we want to improve our endurance and tone our muscles, we exercise with light weights and high repetitions. We define high repetitions as exceeding 12 repetitions.

Bodybuilders develop specialized programs. They lift five or six times per week and dedicate each workout to one or two muscle groups. For example, one workout focuses on the chest. Thus, they do five different types of chest exercises with a minimum of three repetitions each. Then they exercise the back the next day, while the legs on the third. Of course, bodybuilders rarely engage in aerobic exercise since aerobic exercise consumes some of the muscles for energy.

This chapter's critical point is that aerobic and anaerobic exercises are great for a person's health but may not help them lose weight. Furthermore, exercise may not prevent health problems. For example, the health guru James Fuller Fixx jump-started the fitness revolution in America by writing the bestseller – *The Complete Book of Running*. Unfortunately, he died of a heart attack at 52 while jogging from blocked arteries feeding his heart. He had severe atherosclerosis and fatty deposits in the arteries. Atherosclerosis restricts blood flow through the arteries and, in severe cases, will block the blood flow. (It seems heart disease strikes many men around age 50 [287].) Therefore, exercise and fasting complement each other. Exercise strengthens the body, while fasting helps repair the body and keeps it in top shape.

Bariatric Surgery

Some obese people go for bariatric surgery when all other weight loss measures fail. Bariatric refers to the branch of medicine that deals with obesity, while bariatric surgery involves a variety of operations performed on the stomach. The overweight and obese choose which surgery they want. For the least invasive surgery, surgeons place a silicon balloon in the patient's stomach and fill it with a sterile liquid. The balloon occupies volume and reduces the food the stomach can hold. Other techniques involve a surgeon wrapping a lap band around the upper portion of the stomach to shrink it. Finally, the morbidly obese with a BMI exceeding 40% can opt for gastric bypass surgery, which is the most invasive surgery. A surgeon staples the stomach to make it smaller and then reroutes and shortens the small intestines.

Bariatric surgery shrinks the patients' stomachs and, thus, forces the patients to reduce their caloric intake. The patients will become nauseous or will vomit if they overeat [11].

Of course, the patients lose massive amounts of weight after bariatric surgery. The lap band group lost 20.0% of their body weight after two years and experienced a drop in their triglycerides and blood glucose levels [288]. Their HDL cholesterol also increased compared to the control group [288]. Finally, 43% of the patients witnessed a remission of Type 2 diabetes [288].

Gastric bypass surgery is the most invasive surgery and causes the most weight loss, 38% [289]. In ten days, patients lost 8.69 pounds (or 3.95 kg) and shaved 1.68 from their BMI [290]. Finally, 83% of the patients with diabetes went into remission [290]. Thus, bariatric surgery cured patients of diabetes from severe restriction of their eating habits.

Bariatric surgery works because it restores the hormonal balance in the patients. Patients with Type 2 diabetes improve before the weight comes off [11, 290]. Thus, it provides evidence that the hormonal imbalance causes obesity and not vice versa. The surgery also does not slow down the patients' metabolism, which curses dieters by restricting their caloric intake [11]. The patients also feel satiated since little food fills the stomach [290].

Bariatric surgery is not cheap. The lap band surgery costs as low as \$15,000, while stomach stapling costs around \$25,000 [291]. The cost depends on the hospital and surgery type. Gastric bypass surgery permanently modifies the body, while banding and gastric balloons are easily reversed. For the balloon the surgeon pops the balloon and removes it from the stomach. Hence, the surgery does not modify the body.

Some Americans visit Mexico for bariatric surgery and pay bargain prices between \$3,500 and \$10,000. (Ironically, bariatric surgery costs the same in Malaysia.) As we say here in Malaysia, a Chinese iPhone is a Chinese iPhone. We think we found a bargain, but then we have nothing but problems with the phone. Several victims of Mexican butcher doctors posted videos on YouTube about their horror stories of their bargain surgeries. Typically, the consumer gets what he or she pays for - buyer beware!

Some patients experience complications from bariatric surgery and require additional surgery. Furthermore, a patient may need an adjustment to his or her band, or the patient's esophagus narrows. Then the patient has trouble eating. The surgeon must install a large tube to expand the esophagus [11].

Ironically, fasting does not cost a penny, does not modify the body, and shares many of the health benefits of bariatric surgery. Of course, fasting is probably the last thing patients would consider doing, even though it should be at the top of the list.

We should note that fasting and bariatric surgery are not compatible. During the feasting cycle, the patient must eat plenty of food to ensure the body has the minimum required nutrients. However, bariatric surgery limits food intake. Unfortunately, mixing fasting and bariatric surgery could lead to gradual starvation over time.

9. The Backlash against Fasting

"Are you nuts?"

– My best friend

The quote, "Are you nuts?" comes from my best friend of 40 years. I told him that I fasted twice a week and had just finished a 30-hour fast. In addition, a bodybuilder told me I was crazy to fast for 30 hours, although he fasts intermittently for 18 hours once per week. Thus, everyone holds strong views against fasting, especially for long durations.

Fasting has transformed my life. I receive daily compliments from my colleagues, co-workers, and students. They see the transformation. The change transcends the weight loss. People compliment how good my skin looks and how much younger and healthier I look. They see me gorge at the gatherings. For example, one day, we celebrated a colleague's birthday. I ate five slices of pizza, drank four cups of soda, and ate a large slice of chocolate cake. I even scooped up and ate the extra frosting and cake crumbs from the cake platter. I noticed everyone else avoided the soda and ate a small slice of cake. They acted like the chocolate cake hid black scorpions ready to sting them.

People always want to know the secret to my weight loss and transformation. Some of them also struggle to lose weight. Then I tell them my secret – I fast twice weekly for at least 24 hours. I get the blank stares as if I were passing out Bibles at an Ozzy Osbourne concert. I even tell them I can eat anything I want during my feasting days. Nope. No conversions. Just blank stares like I just ripped a thunderous fart, and everyone pretends not to smell it.

My Malaysian Chinese girlfriend, Alice, has witnessed the transformation and weight loss. She knows I fast and worries I will leave her for another woman. Several times, I tried to convince her to fast with me. However, she says she needs the energy to do work. I once explained to her that the body stores fat and that fat provides energy. Wow, that conversation did not go well. For the good news, she did not make me walk home. Boy, that would have been a long walk home. However, I have convinced Alice to fast for 16 hours several times. She needs a little more persuasion.

Fasting freaks people out. Thus, in this chapter, we examine fasting from the viewpoints of the medical establishment, the food industry, and the government. Finally, we debunk most of the fasting myths.

The Medical Establishment

In the United States, medical doctors are hostile towards fasting. They act like a person will go into a diabetic coma if they do not eat something every two hours.

We visit doctors and expect them to be masters of human health. For chubby patients, doctors give the same advice to lose weight— exercise more, eat more fruits and vegetables, and avoid fats. I heard this speech numerous times, ad nauseam. Then Dr. Fung once wrote that medical doctors receive little training in nutrition [11]. For instance, Dr. Fung says he had about four hours of lectures on nutrition out of his nine years of medical education and training [11].

The top medical schools in the United States include Harvard University, John Hopkins, and the Mayo Clinic. Medical students study human anatomy, science, substance abuse, and end-of-life care, but there is no class in nutrition. Hence, nutrition would fall as a subtopic in one of the courses. However, I face the same problem when I teach my students finance. I have three years to teach them and want to know if I am preparing them for the real business world.

The hostility of medical doctors is nothing new; it existed in the early 1900s. Upton Sinclair wrote about the doctors' attitude in his book. In Sinclair's time, doctors created ointments, potions, and concoctions in their backroom labs and sold them directly to patients [1]. In addition, Dr. Edward Dewey wrote about how intermittent fasting had cured various ailments and illnesses and wrote a famous book – *The No Breakfast Plan and the Fasting–Cure* [2]. The *British Medical Journal* scoffed called his evidence a "foolish delusion." We still possess this mentality today, but the pharmaceutical industry creates new concoctions. Then the doctors prescribe the medicines to their patients.

The healthcare industry holds the view that a sick person must take a pill to make the person well again, or the sick person needs surgery where the doctors cut into the body to remove or modify the tissues. Medicines and surgery are costly in the United States. The doctors, medical establishments, and pharmaceutical companies reap enormous profits on the other side of the accounting equation.

If we are savvy business people with a sliver of conscience and want to make money, how could we extract the most money from the customers? First, if we make a one-time sale, we want to provide a product or service that will cost substantial money. We want to sell the customer a decked-out Cadillac Escalade with gold-plated rims and a smooth leather interior. Let us remember the sound system that will rattle and shake all the windows in the neighborhood as we stroll by in style. The second way to drain the customers is the customer returns every month to keep buying that product or service. That is precisely what the healthcare industry does to enrich itself.

Hospitals make their big money from surgery. For example, heart bypass surgery is a joint surgery where doctors take a blood vessel from one part of the body and reroute a blocked artery that feeds the heart. Americans are willing to pay a high price for this service because heart disease is America's number one killer. Unfortunately, 697,000 Americans died from heart disease in 2020.

Bypass surgery costs between $70,000 and $200,000 depending on the hospital and whether the patient suffered additional complications [292]. Some patients require physical therapy and medications for additional costs. Dr. Fuhrman says heart bypass surgery rarely extends life [9]. However, it does not stop the patients from cashing in all their assets to get one. I would not hesitate to cash in all my assets for surgery if a doctor convinced me that I needed one. God only gave us one life in this world, and we cannot take the assets with us.

The pharmaceutical industry fulfills the second criterion to make money by selling medicine monthly to patients. Moreover, business is good. The pharmaceutical industry patents its concoctions. A patent grants the company the exclusive right to produce its concoction for 20 years in the United States. Another company can only produce that product if it receives permission from the patent holder. Otherwise, the patent holder can sue for patent infringement.

A patent grants monopoly power. Monopolies charge the highest price and sell the lowest quantity compared to all market structures. On the other hand, a competitive market sells for the lowest price and sells the highest quantity. Do not get me wrong. I am not against patents because companies must invest billions of dollars to finance research and development. Furthermore, patents allow companies to recoup their research and development costs, but sometimes, companies go overboard on prescription drug prices.

Prescriptions, even the cheap ones, are profitable. For example, people in the early stages of diabetes take Metformin, the 7th most prescribed drug in the United States in 2017 [293]. The Centers for Disease Control and Prevention estimates that 30.3 million Americans have diabetes [294]. Hence, if people with diabetes pay $8 per one-month supply of Metformin [293], and 10 million diabetics take Metformin every year, that means the pharmaceutical industry earns $960 million yearly (or $8x12x10 million) in revenue. That is a tad under a billion yearly.

We see the paradox of modern medicine. The medicine treats the symptoms but never cures the patients. As Dr. Fuhrman learned in medical school, all medications and drugs are toxic to the body [9]. Medicines and drugs do not provide nutrients or energy. Instead, they interfere with the body's natural processes [9]. Thus, the medications help alleviate the symptoms but ensure the medicines never cure us. That way, we can keep buying medicines monthly for the rest of our lives. Hence, we have a paradox.

Hence, we identified a problem with fasting. Companies cannot patent fasting, while fasting requires no medicines or potions. In addition, medical doctors advise against fasting. For example, we go to a doctor who recommends that we water fast for two days. Then the miraculous healing power of fasting cures us. Next time we get sick, we stay home fast and do not bother to see the doctor again. The next thing we know, the doctor is knocking on our door and begging us to buy a $2,000 vacuum cleaner. Fasting on a large scale can severely affect the medical industry.

The Food Industry

We expect the food industry to oppose fasting. The food industry does not make money if we do not eat. For example, a person fasts twice a week for 24 hours, which means the person fasts from one dinner to the next the following day, from breakfast to breakfast or lunch to lunch. Thus, that person misses two meals for one fast and four meals per week for two fasts. If that person spends $10 on a meal and fasts intermittently the whole year, they save $2,080 annually. That means the food companies see a decline of $2,080. Now imagine the financial hardship fasting would cause if millions of people started intermittent fasting.

The dynamics are complicated. Some fasters alter their buying behavior when they see they save money. They could purchase better quality food. For example, when I go shopping, I buy more expensive food because I know I save some money from fasting when not eating. The high-quality food has an upside. I love the taste of food when I break a fast. Thus, I want the good stuff. Also, fasters tend to overeat for their first meal after breaking the fast.

Another dynamic is a faster lifespan. A faster could live longer, so they eat for a longer lifetime. Using the exact numbers, fasting twice weekly yields 17 meals per week. We assume the person eats three meals daily except for the fasting period. That person would eat about $8,840 yearly. If that faster lives an additional 10 years, the food industry would reap $88,400. Unfortunately, many companies in the United States are geared to earn short-run profits.

The food industry would not benefit if many people began fasting in the short run. The food industry is one of the most competitive industries in the United States and has a small profit margin. Consequently, a slight decrease in food demand in the short run could bankrupt companies. Thus, we expect the food industry to oppose fasting.

The Government

The U.S. or state governments will likely refrain from jumping on board and advocating fasting. The answer is simple. Retirees stop working and stop contributing tax revenue to the government. Instead, they receive money from Social Security and begin cashing in their retirement plans. Americans could start collecting Social Security benefits as early as 62. Although the government reduces the benefits for retiring early, retirees can receive full benefits for retiring between 67 and 70 years of age, depending on when they were born [295].

Men, on average, live until 76.3 years, while women lived until 81.1 years in 2015 [147]. Men and women could collect 10 years of Social Security before they die. What would happen if many retired Americans adopted intermittent fasting and started living healthily until they were 120? Now, the government would pay 50 years in social security benefits. The Social Security Administration would bankrupt faster than rain falling from the heavens. Technically, a federal agency cannot go bankrupt, but a cash flow crisis would cripple operations. Then the crisis spreads to the pensioners dependent on their monthly social security checks.

Society would need to restructure if people lived until 120 years old. That means a person could work for one employer for 100 years. Only the devil can devise such a 100-year servitude.

Fasting on a large scale would evoke another problem. Many Americans suffer from medical problems and take a large variety of medicines. The immense demand for healthcare has inflated the industry to $3 trillion annually [296]. That is a large chunk of the U.S. economy, at least 15%. What if a large portion of Americans started fasting and became healthy? The healthcare industry would crumble and start shedding jobs.

The healthcare industry employs doctors and nurses who have spent a lifetime learning their skills. Medical doctors must complete a bachelor's degree, four years of medical school, and between three and seven years of residency to apply for a medical license. Furthermore, nurses require at least a four-year degree. However, many nurses complete a master's and additional training, with additional training equating to higher salaries. Thus, fasting on a large scale could lead to massive job losses for highly educated people who expected to earn lucrative salaries.

We expect the politicians to hear the doctors' and nurses' plight. The politicians need to be re-elected to continue their jobs. The politicians pay millions in campaign costs to work a job that pays a fraction of campaign costs. For example, Congressmen and Senators earned $174,000 annually in Congress in 2017, while election costs exceeded $3 million. It would not be smart for Congressmen to pay campaign costs out of their pocket. Thus, other people pay campaign costs, explaining why politicians always cave into public demands and bend backward to their financial contributors.

Hospitals, insurance companies, pharmaceutical companies, and the food industry are large contributors to political campaigns. Yes, the companies buy votes. Politicians know that if they vote against a financial backer, that financial backer will contribute to the opposition in the next election. That is why we get politicians who talk on both sides of their mouths at all levels of government. The healthcare and food industries would be hostile towards fasting so that the politicians would be hostile.

If fasting were to become popular, we would expect the government to use its authority and power to go after the people who advocated it. For instance, the state arrested and charged Dr. Shelton and many associates several times for practicing medicine without a license [149]. Dr. Shelton never prescribed medications or performed surgical operations. He opened several medical clinics and supervised thousands of fasts. However, state governments viewed him as a criminal and ordered the police to arrest him.

The Soviet Union

Researchers and corporations may neglect fasting since the corporation cannot patent the fasting process. Patents cover devices or chemicals and not processes. The goal is to make money, encouraging scientists and researchers to search for drugs and medicines to extend life. They file a patent with the U.S. Trademark and Patent Office that grants the patent holder 20 years as the exclusive producer. That way, the company charges high prices and squeezes customers for everything they have for a lifesaving drug.

Thus, fasting cannot be patented and provides little financial awards in studying it.

Some researchers study fasting, but we cannot predict how much future research they will conduct. I am also a researcher in finance and renewable energy. Our academic careers depend on publishing papers in good journals and obtaining research grants. Researchers studying fasting may need help getting grants since corporations offer grants for future products and patents. Often, governments mirror the corporations and provide grants for tangible results. Consequently, researchers pursue research to boost careers, reputations, and salaries, but not necessarily to further human knowledge.

We, of course, must be careful of research funded by a grant. A research grant could bias experiments and research. Remember that old idiom – do not bite the hand that feeds you.

Times could change. Iranian academics established *The Journal of Nutrition, Fasting, and Health* in 2013. The journal, published in English, covers all aspects of fasting, and anyone can download articles for free. Unfortunately, the hostile relations between Iran and the United States could prevent researchers and scientists in the West from reading the Iranian journal. Believe it or not, only one country in modern history has studied fasting on a large scale: the Soviet Union.

It seems odd to discuss the Soviet Union in a fasting book. The Soviet Union was a murderous state where millions disappeared under Stalin when the infamous secret police knocked on troubler makers' doors at midnight. Furthermore, Stalin starved millions of people in the USSR when the state confiscated the livestock and restructured all industries in the Soviet Union.

The Soviet Union created two privileged classes. The first class consisted of members of the communist party who drove cars, lived in the best apartments, and shopped at their exclusive stores with fully stocked shelves. We should not be surprised. The communist party members were the politicians. Of course, they lived well compared to the people they ruled over. Then the scientists and professors filled the second privileged class. Consequently, the Soviet Union excelled in mathematics and physical sciences. The

Soviet Union put the first man, Yuri Gagarin, into outer space, which sparked the space race between the United States and the Soviet Union.

The scientists in the Soviet Union studied fasting as a medical cure. Dr. Uri Nickolayev discovered fasting as a cure for schizophrenia accidentally [28]. The story begins with a schizophrenic patient refusing to eat. Instead of forcing the patient to eat food, Dr. Nickolayev let him be. Surprisingly, the symptoms of schizophrenia disappeared after two weeks of not eating food. That piqued the doctor's curiosity. Then Dr. Nickolayev started conducting water fasts in the Moscow Psychiatric Institute to cure patients [28].

The patients water fasted for 20 to 30 days [289]. They must drink a minimum of one liter of water daily and exercise three hours daily, including outdoor walks [28]. The patients breathed fresh air while the sunlight hit their skin. They also practiced breathing exercises, afternoon naps, massages, showers, and cleansing enemas [28]. Ironically, fasting resorts follow the same guidelines, including yoga and tai chi, but charge premium prices.

The fasting treatment cured 64% of people with schizophrenia, and 47% of patients maintained their improvement over six years [28]. When the hospital discharged patients, doctors conducted periodic home checks on the patients for 10 years [28]. People with schizophrenia usually have abnormal buildups of protein in the brain. The patients would periodically fast for short periods at home to remove the protein buildup [28]. Alzheimer's is another disease with an abnormal accumulation of proteins in the brain that fasting may help alleviate.

Dr. Nickolayev expanded fasting to manic-depressives [28], overweight teenagers [297], people afflicted with cardiovascular diseases [297], and alcoholics [28]. If the alcoholics continue to drink after the fast, they greatly reduce their consumption [28] because their bodies become more sensitive to alcohol. Ironically, doctors would not treat cancer patients with fasting [28], even though we already learned in this book that fasting reduces or eliminates some cancers.

Dr. Nickolayev notified the Soviet Academy of Sciences. Although the academy was skeptical at first, it dedicated resources, doctors, and scientists to studying water fasts. The intellectuals of the Soviet Union took the study of fasting seriously.

With the breakup of the Soviet Union, fasting lost its popularity because Russian doctors recommended medical supervision of fasters. Most Russians cannot afford to pay for medical supervision. In places like Siberia, medical doctors still practice fasting. On the other hand, Russian fasting resorts attract health tourists. Several resorts in the Russian wilderness cost half as much as the fasting resorts in Europe [297].

The Soviet Union had many intelligent people running the system, so why did the system fail? We have a simple answer. The bureaucrats made all economic decisions. They decided how much the factories would charge, how much to produce, how much labor to use, etc. A person needed permission from the government for every tiny thing. For example, a person living in a village needed a particular document to relocate and work in a city. Sometimes, a village guy would marry a city girl to get that document. Yes, the bureaucracies were that anal. When I lived there in the mid-1990s, the bureaucracies were a headache unless one tucked a couple of Benjamins inside the documents. (I visited places where Americans were not viewed highly, but I never had trouble buying with American dollars.)

The Soviet Union grew phenomenally during the 1960s, but severe shortages and degradation set in in the 1980s. The bureaucrats also froze technology, and the Soviet Union fell behind Western nations. Then the system collapsed in 1991.

Myths of Fasting

In this section, we debunk several myths about fasting.

> **Myth #1** – Breakfast is the day's most important meal [143].

We have heard this saying since birth. As soon as we rise, we must eat to keep that metabolism burning energy like shoveling coal into a steam locomotive to keep the train going. Schools insist that every student must have breakfast to perform well academically. In one study of healthy adults, the participants did not suffer from mental decline after two days of severe calorie deprivation [298]. Of course, it makes sense. If missing a few meals caused a severe mental decline, we would have never survived as a species in the wild.

For many people, including me, breakfast is the smallest meal of the day and the most leisurely meal to miss, even though people have not eaten since yesterday's dinner. How can the smallest and easiest meal to miss be the most important?

Dr. Edward Dewey wrote a popular book in 1900 that recommended that his patients and sick people refrain from breakfast daily [2]. The fasters could still enjoy their coffee or tea in the morning [2]. He described the numerous ailments and sicknesses intermittent fasting had cured. If our bodies need breakfast, shouldn't our bodies weaken, while our ailments and sickness strengthen?

The myth has even spread to Malaysia. I heard one commercial on a popular radio station with young people espousing the importance of eating breakfast in the morning.

> **Myth #2** – East small, frequent meals or snacks to boost metabolism and stabilize blood sugar [12, 143].

American society has changed eating habits as we have become a nation of snackers. Every day, Americans eat five or six times daily [11, 12]. We have a false notion that men and women must always eat. Thus, six small meals are always better than three large ones. However, the evidence suggests no difference between gorging and nibbling on the human body if we eat the same calories throughout the day [279, 280]. Please note that the studies omit fasting and the potential to gorge on one massive daily meal.

I remember growing up in the 1970s in Michigan. At school and home, we ate three meals with no snacking between meals. I was lucky to get a glass of milk in the afternoon before supper, but the snacking lifestyle crept into college. I gorged at the university's cafeterias and snacked on chips, soda, and candy between meals. Thus, snacking caused me to eat more calories during the day. Then

I gained the freshmen 10, when first-year students gain 10 pounds (4.55kg) during their first semester in college.

I turned into a snacker. For example, I copied the eating habits of the bodybuilders at my gym, where the bodybuilders eat six small meals daily. I reduced my caloric intake by eating frequently, and the frequent eating would ward off the hunger pangs. However, this notion needs to be corrected. Since I always consumed carbohydrates, I kept my insulin levels high throughout the day, while my digestive system only rested briefly at night. The frequent eating turned my body into a carbohydrate-burning machine, not a fat-burning one.

When I started 30-hour fasts twice per week, I stopped snacking. I can quickly go six hours without eating on my feasting days. Eating is psychological. If I can go 30 hours without eating on a fasting day, then six hours between meals is nothing. I also eat until I feel satiated.

I go out of my way to prevent snacking. For instance, I drink my cappuccino or latte within an hour of breakfast or lunch. That way, I include coffee as a meal, not a snack. Then I drink tea without sugar and cream between meals.

> **Myth #3** – The body consumes muscle and not fat during fasts [11].

This myth may be true. The body ramps up the production of the human growth hormone, which helps spare the breakdown of muscle tissue. However, the bodybuilders at my gym and the scientific literature support the view that fasters lose some muscle mass. Dr. Shelton reported that skeletal muscles lose up to 40% of their weight during a fast [3]. A person does not lose muscle cells per se. Instead, the muscle cells become smaller as the person loses fat and glycogen stored in the muscles [3]. In addition, several studies indicated a loss of muscle mass because the liver manufactures glucose from amino acids with muscles being a source [9, 17, 23, 24]. The red blood cells and liver require glucose for energy, while the brain needs at least 25% glucose.

The body's attack on muscles depends on the person. As people's bodies ramp up the consumption of ketones for fuel, their bodies spare protein. Women and lean individuals switch to burning ketones at a faster rate than men and the obese [17]. Thus, women and lean individuals could lose less muscle than their counterparts, which is unfair.

I talked to the bodybuilders at my gym. The bodybuilders appreciate fasting and believe it provides many health benefits. However, they avoid fasting before competitions because they claim they lost 22 pounds (or 10 kg), which is a fantastic weight loss. They believe they lost between 13.2 and 15.4 pounds (or 6 and 7 kg) of fat and between 6.6 and 8.8 pounds (or 3 and 4 kg) of muscle.

Fasters may lose some muscle tissue from the fast because fasting restores balance to the human body. For instance, bodybuilders overly develop their massive physiques and large muscles, which become abnormal. Large bulky muscles could pose a detriment in the long run, especially if the person no longer needs these large muscles. Thus, the body consumes the nonvital tissues first because the body can quickly rebuild these tissues during a feasting cycle. A little muscle loss during fasting is beneficial to help the body shed unneeded muscles and rebuild them when needed.

Muscle loss is not a big deal. Exercise helps complement the benefits of fasting. We use resistance and weight training to strengthen and build muscles and aerobic exercise to strengthen our cardiovascular system. Hence, we have an incentive to renew our gym membership.

➢ **Myth #4** – Fasting slows metabolism.

To be healthy, functioning humans, we must burn energy to support our life processes. Our lungs need energy to breathe. The brain consumes energy to think and send and receive signals from all parts of our body. The heart consumes energy to pump blood to and from all cells. The liver and digestive system require energy to break down food into energy, minerals, and vitamins. We refer to this collective energy consumption to support life our metabolism, which we also call the basal metabolic rate.

Metabolism is our body's thermostat. As teenagers, we could trek outside in the snow in a t-shirt and shorts and not shiver. Our metabolism was high, and we could eat anything and everything without gaining an ounce of fat. As we age, we shiver in the breeze on a warm spring day. Our metabolism slows, and we begin eating less. Then it is like we glance at food, and our bodies start piling on the weight.

Since the last century, we have known that restricting food consumption reduces metabolism [9, 11, 12, 273]. For example, if we reduce our food intake by 10%, our body gradually lowers the thermostat, causing the metabolism to slow down by about 10% [12]. Thus, people lose weight on a calorie-restricted diet, but the weight loss slows and eventually reaches a plateau. Eventually, the dieter resumes standard eating patterns because he or she always feels hungry, cold, and lethargic. Then the dieter regains the weight rapidly.

Conversely, fasting boosts metabolism by 3% [10-12]. The metabolism remains high as long as we break our fasts within two days and resume normal eating.

> **Myth #5** – Fasting leads to low blood sugar or hypoglycemia [11].

Symptoms of low blood sugar include feeling shaky, nervous, sweating, clamminess, and chills. People with diabetes know the signs well as they quickly drink a glass of orange juice or eat a sugary snack to counteract low sugar levels. Death results if the blood sugar level drops too low.

People worry that fasting will cause low blood sugar. However, the body regulates blood sugar well. During a fast, most cells switch to burning ketones for fuel. Although the red blood cells, liver, and 25% of the brain's energy require glucose, the liver can produce glucose from amino acids from the muscles. The liver can also make glucose from glycerol, which comes from the breakdown of triglycerides, i.e., fat [3, 11, 17].

People with diabetes must be careful during fasts because they experience wide swings in their blood sugar levels. Consequently, a medical doctor should supervise them during a fast to ensure their blood sugar levels vary little.

> **Myth #6** – Fasting starves the person [11].

We discussed this issue in the first chapter. A person performs a fast correctly if the body uses nonvital tissues and cells as fuel. During a fast, the body utilizes fat stores, possibly some muscle protein, and the recycled proteins and substances from autophagy and apoptosis. The body causes a cell to kill itself via apoptosis if it is damaged or old, i.e., senescent.

A faster enters starvation by prolonging the fast too long or is highly malnourished. A person will not likely starve on a two-day fast. For instance, a person weighing 200 pounds (or 90.9 kg) with 20% body fat has 40 pounds (or 18.2 kg) of fat. The fat reserves easily power the body for 40 days or more.

The fasting duration depends on a person's fat reserves. The longest-known fast comes from a Scottish man, Angus Barbieri [299]. He started his fast, weighing 455.4 pounds (or 207 kg), and fasted for one year and 17 days in 1965 [299, 300]. He lost 275 pounds (or 125 kg) [299], which equaled 0.72 pounds (or 0.33 kg) daily. He drank black coffee, black tea, and water and took a multivitamin, potassium, sodium, and yeast supplements daily [299, 300]. Yeast resembles spirulina and contains the nine essential amino acids and the vitamin B complexes. The body uses vitamin Bs in cell metabolism, energy burning, and brain function. A doctor monitored Angus's fast and recorded no medical complications [299, 300].

As long as the faster has plenty of fat reserves, he or she will not starve during a fast.

> **Myth #7** – Fasting causes overeating [11, 12].

This myth does contain a kernel of truth. People who fast intermittently for two days or less tend to overeat during their first meal [12]. However, the fasters do not replace all the calories they had missed during a fast. They usually eat 30% more calories during the first meal [238]. Then normal eating patterns resume.

People doing prolonged fasts of three days or more must transition to eating food again. Their first meals are juices, broths, soups, fruits, and vegetables. Consequently, the fasters are not likely to overeat during their first meals because they will experience extreme discomfort. The digestive system requires an adjustment time to begin processing food again.

> **Myth #8** – Fasting starves the body of nutrients [11, 12].

We know this myth is false. People usually fast for two weeks or more. They look younger and have more energy, while their health problems disappear and their muscles become stronger. If fasters are deprived of nutrients, then fasters would see and feel the deprivation. They would look sick after a fast if the fast had caused nutrient deficiencies. For example, vitamin C deficiency causes scurvy, while vitamin D and calcium deficiencies cause bone problems.

As a marvelous machine, the body reduces waste to a minimum during a fast [3]. The body conserves vitamins and minerals like calcium, sodium, potassium, and magnesium [3, 12]. We must remember that we quickly utilize the resources we have eaten in the past. All we are doing is rummaging in the back of the cupboard for old cans of soups and vegetables. Fasting helps us use the old cans of food that our bodies stored long ago.

> **Myth #9** – Fasting collapses the heart within six days [3].

This funny myth dates from the beginning of the 20th century. Doctors warned potential fasters that their hearts would collapse within six days of fasting [3]. Furthermore, Upton Sinclair (1911) conversed with a well-known, respected physician who refused to believe a man or woman could survive beyond five days without nourishment [1].

We know this myth is false. Angus Barbieri fasted for one year and 17 days. In addition, a healthy, normal-weighing man or woman can fast for a month and still have plenty of fat reserves left over.

The doctors perpetuated a false myth to scare patients away from fasting.

"Fasting is the greatest remedy, the physician within."

– Paracelsus

I need help with healthy eating. Although I eat plenty of fast food, along with decadent iced coffees, ice cream, and chocolate, I also eat some fresh fruit and vegetables. Thus, I give the reader tips and recipes that maximize healthy eating because we need nutritious meals to ensure our bodies have all the necessary vitamins and minerals to endure a fast.

My favorite salads are raw, delicious, and filled with garlic and onions. I eat them regularly and drink the leftover sour brine.

Tips on Healthy Eating

We should cook most of our meals at home. Restaurants and grocery stores compete in a competitive market and earn profit margins between 3 and 5%. Therefore, every penny counts. When they prepare food, they gravitate towards the cheapest ingredients. At home, we control what we put in our food.

> ➤ **Tip #49:** Always add fresh vegetables and fruits to dishes instead of things that come from a can. Just read the nutritional information on the side of the can or box. Canned fruits and vegetables are nutritionally dead because the processing and cooking destroy many vitamins and antioxidants. Thus, we take the extra 15 minutes to dice some fresh fruits and vegetables. We can also add frozen fruits and vegetables because the freezing helps retain their nutrients.

From my experience in the kitchen, seasonings, and meat are the two most essential ingredients we must use. A cheap seasoning has a bland, dull taste and adds a minuscule flavor. Cheap meats are tough, dry hockey pucks, while cheap ground beef breaks into an oily, gelatinous gristle that ruins the meal. That leads to our next tip.

> **Tip #50:** Buy better ingredients. I always go for the omega-three enriched eggs at the supermarket. Of course, I trust the farmers that they have fed the chickens flax seeds.

Fresh herbs and seasonings add flavor to a dish. For example, when I make spaghetti sauce, I simmer freshly diced tomatoes, onions, garlic, and seasonings. I add tomato paste to thicken the sauce. Many people comment on my spaghetti sauce, especially when I add fresh oregano, basil, and thyme. I can even freeze the sauce in plastic containers for future meals.

My church has a potluck lunch after service. The church members usually devour my dish. Adding fresh herbs to a dish enhances the flavor, which leads to the next tip.

> **Tip #51:** Many herbs, such as basil, oregano, and thyme, can grow in containers or like weeds in the garden. Fresh herbs add flavor to a dish and impart many health benefits.

Home remedies often include garlic and onions because they have potent medicinal properties. Of course, the Asian home remedies also add ginger to the mix. Eating copious amounts of garlic and onions helps prolong life. For instance, my grandmother made it to 85, although she had diabetes, heart disease, obesity, and high blood pressure for 40 years. She always ate garlic and onions, raw or cooked, with everything. She was also a stubborn woman. I also believe she lived a long time to anger her doctors. She outlived most of them.

Many people avoid garlic and onions because the odor emanates from our sweat pores and breath. However, the health and longevity benefits far exceed the attractiveness to the opposite sex. That is why we have mouthwash, breath mints, cologne, and perfume.

I always stock my kitchen with garlic, onions, and shallots that I can quickly dice within minutes and sprinkle into any meal.

> **Tip #52:** When a recipe calls for garlic or onions, at least double or triple the garlic and onions. Chef Emeril is onto something when kicking up the garlic another notch.

Another good ingredient is extra virgin and light olive oil, which is used in cooking and salads. Light olive oil means the producers removed polyphenols and impurities, giving the olive oil a lighter appearance. I use both oils to sauté food or eggs at the lowest stove heat because olive oil has a low smoke point. Hence, cooking meat at medium or high heat levels burns the oil and ruins the dish with a burnt smell. We must switch oils to sear meat or cook at medium heat or higher.

> **Tip #53:** We should substitute light olive oil instead of vegetable oils. Many claim olive oil is healthier than vegetable oils and better for the heart because olive oil contains omega-3 fatty acids. Meanwhile, vegetable oils are saturated with omega-6 fatty acids [12]. Although our bodies need both fatty acids, too much omega-6 causes inflammation [12]. Almost all processed foods use cheap vegetable oils filled with omega-6 fatty acids to reduce costs.

Olive oil is an expensive oil. The producers harvest the olives and use a press to extract the olive oil from the crushed olives. Some shifty producers use heat and chemicals to remove every minuscule drop of olive oil and may even add vegetable oil and green coloring and sell the olive oil as pure extra virgin olive oil. When I make one of my cold salads with olive oil, pure olive oil congeals in the refrigerator. On the other hand, olive oils adulterated with vegetable oils do not solidify in the fridge.

Another culprit in Americans' declining health is their high sugar consumption. Sugar spikes the insulin level, causing the cells to utilize glucose for energy. The high insulin level causes our bodies to store more fat.

When I eat high levels of sugar, my taste buds dull. On several occasions, I reduced my sugar consumption as much as possible, hoping to lose some weight. In the absence of sugar, my taste buds became super sensitive; I could even taste the sugar in white bread. Do not get me wrong; I still eat sugar but reduce my consumption.

The key is moderation. For example, when I bake cookies and cakes for the church, I reduce the sugar by about 30%. The cakes and cookies still taste great, but we can also savor the other ingredients. I also use real butter and brown sugar, and the church members scarf down my cookies and cakes as if they have not eaten in weeks.

> ➤ **Tip #54:** Reduce sugar consumption. The key is moderation. I have started experimenting with stevia, a natural sweetener in my recipes. The keto diet offers many delicious snacks sweetened with stevia, erythritol, and monk fruit. Stevia and monk fruit are natural.

We should avoid high-fructose corn syrup (HFCS). Some researchers and doctors claim that consuming too much fructose causes fatty liver, insulin resistance, and elevated triglycerides [12, 260]. A diet high in fructose could increase the risk of obesity, diabetes, and heart disease [260].

We should not eliminate all fructose. Fruits contain fructose along with fiber, vitamins, and minerals. Furthermore, table sugar contains 50% fructose and 50% glucose. Every cell in the body can utilize glucose, while only the liver can process fructose [12, 260]. Again, we have returned to reducing sugar consumption again.

The bad news is that the food industry puts HFCS in almost all processed food. We can avoid HFCS by cooking more homemade meals.

> ➤ **Tip #55:** Avoid HFCS. Corn contains trace amounts of sugar. Food companies manufacture HFCS from cornstarch.

We should avoid trans-fat in margarine, shortening, and hydrogenated vegetable oils. The food industry artificially produces trans-fat from vegetable oils. For example, vegetable oils are unsaturated, meaning they share chemical bonds. The problem is that unsaturated oil breaks down and degrades over time [12].

However, the food industry discovered that passing hydrogen through vegetable oil could saturate all the chemical bonds, making the oil chemically stable. Thus, each free bond has a hydrogen atom.

Consequently, the food industry fries food in oil or incorporates trans fat into processed food for extended shelf life. That is the problem. Trans fat does not exist in nature. Trans fat raises LDL cholesterol, the bad cholesterol, and lowers HDL cholesterol, the good cholesterol.

> ➤ **Tip #56:** Avoid trans-fat that we would find in shortening, margarine, and hydrogenated vegetable oils [12].

I live on the Island of Borneo in Malaysia, which has year-round tropical weather. I must keep the kitchen spotless and take the garbage out regularly. If I dice fresh vegetables or fruits, I must immediately put them into Tupperware or the refrigerator. If I leave the fruit and vegetables on the counter, tiny bugs will cover the cutting board and freshly cooked foods within 15 minutes—those little critters even like freshly baked bread. Thus, I must watch freshly cooked bread as it cools. Those little bugs are ravenous.

Here is the thing: If I leave a heavily processed item on the table or counter, like fast food or something made from a box, like hamburger helper or macaroni and cheese, those little critters will not touch it. The exception is table sugar, which I keep in the freezer. The little bugs must know something that we do not or purposely choose to ignore.

I give the readers some good recipes to help them eat more nutritious meals.

Beans

Beans are not just delicious, they are also a powerhouse of nutrition. Rich in plant protein, minerals, B vitamins, and soluble fiber, they are a great addition to any diet. Soluble fiber, in particular, is a hero for our digestive health. It absorbs water in the stomach, slows the absorption of food and sugar, and gives a feeling of fullness. In theory, fiber slows the absorption of glucose and, thus, weakens the insulin response. So, not only are we enjoying a tasty meal, but we're also doing your body a favor.

The problem is beans do not taste good, especially from a can. However, the recipe made from dried beans tastes great. I often start my day with a bowl of homemade beans for breakfast. The recipe comes from my beloved grandmother, a master of Southern cuisine. In the Southern United States, homemade cornbread and beans go together. In Malaysia, I top the beans with a fried egg with a soft golden yolk. Figure 4 shows the recipe for black-eye peas, a dish that always brings back fond memories of family meals.

Figure 4. Black Eye Peas

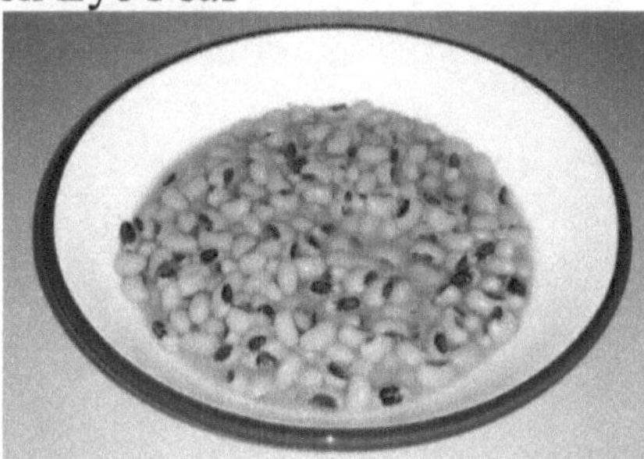

Ingredients
- 1 pound (or 1/2 kilogram) of your favorite beans
- 1/2 pound (1/4 kilogram) beef or pork bones
- 2 bay leaves
- 1 onion, diced
- 2 tablespoons olive oil or butter
- 1 teaspoon sea salt
- 1 teaspoon pepper

Directions

1. Clean and cover beans with water overnight.
2. Simmer beans with bones and bay leaves for 2 to 4 hours on low heat, covered. Pinto and black-eye peas soften quickly, while other beans, such as kidney beans, take longer.

3. Add the remaining ingredients in the last half hour of cooking.

The key to good beans is the bones and oil. These two ingredients make the beans delicious. We feel free to add additional seasonings to our liking.

Bone Broth

We have already discussed the benefits of bone broth, and now it is time to savor its delicious taste. A mug of bone broth is perfect for prolonged fasts beyond 24 hours. Figure 5 shows a picture of the mouthwatering bone broth you're about to make.

Figure 5. Bone Broth

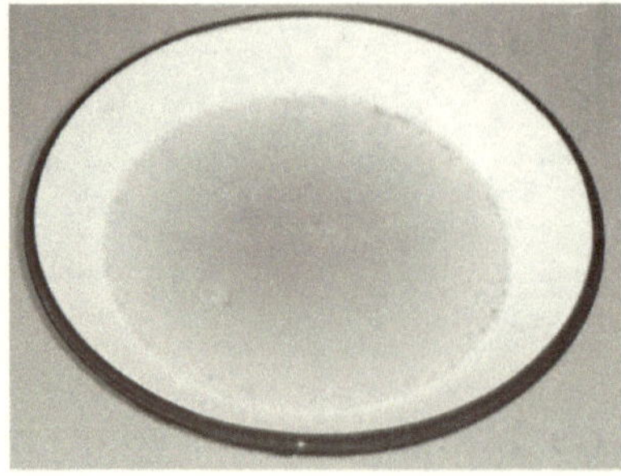

Ingredients
- 1/2 pound (1/4 kilogram) beef, chicken, fish, or pork bones
- 2 bay leaves
- 1 teaspoon sea salt
- 1 teaspoon pepper

Directions

1. Simmer bones and bay leaves at least 3 hours on low heat, covered.
2. Add the salt and pepper in the last half hour of cooking.

Carrot and Cucumber Salad

Carrot-cucumber salad is a favorite in Malaysia at Indian and Muslim restaurants and is shown in Figure 6. I always take a heaping of this salad with fried chicken, curry sauce, and rice.

Figure 6. Carrot-Cucumber Salad

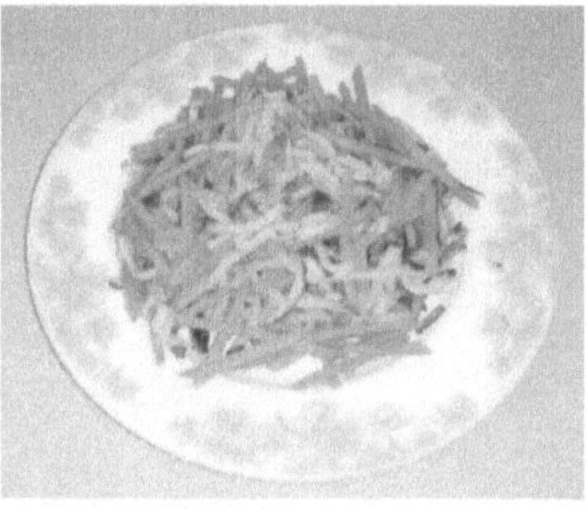

Ingredients
- 1 carrot
- 1 large cucumber
- 2 tablespoons rice or white vinegar
- 2 tablespoons honey
- 1 teaspoon sea salt
- 1 teaspoon pepper

Directions

1. Clean both the carrot and cucumber. Slice the cucumber lengthwise and use a spoon to remove the seed core. Julienne both the carrots and cucumbers. We may adjust the number of carrots and cucumbers to get a ratio of one to one.
2. Julienne, a special shredder from the Asian stores, shreds vegetables into long shoestrings.
3. Mix all ingredients together.

Malaysians offer variations of this dish. Sometimes, they dice and add pineapple or diced spicy chilies.

Carrot Salad

Carrot salad is one of my favorite salads, and I eat it several times each month. I discovered this dish in Central Asia, specifically in the Republic of Kazakhstan, during the mid-1990s. At that time, Kazakhstan was a state of the Soviet Union. Despite the freezing temperatures, I would venture to the open market, braving the cold, to pick up this salad. It was a culinary delight that I still cherish. Figure 7 shows the carrot salad.

Figure 7. Carrot Salad

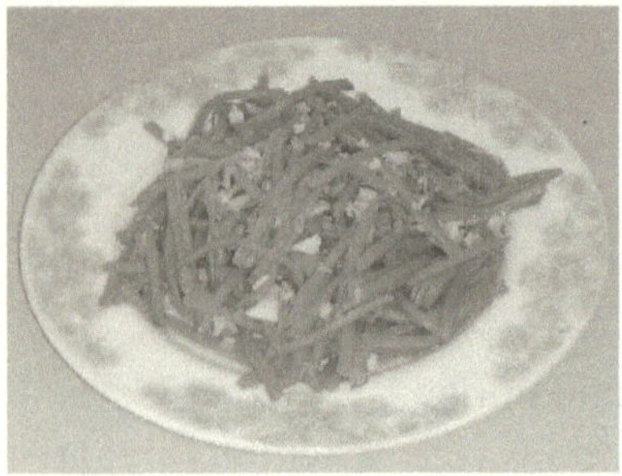

Ingredients
- 3 carrots
- 1/4 cup white vinegar or apple cider vinegar
- 1/4 cup water
- 2 tablespoons honey
- 1/2 teaspoon sea salt
- 1/2 teaspoon black or white pepper
- 3 cloves, finely diced garlic
- 3 shallots finely diced or 1/2 red onion finely diced

Directions

1. Mix the vinegar, water, honey, salt, pepper, shallots, and garlic together. Allow the sauce to absorb the flavors.

2. Julienne the carrots. Julienne is a special shredder, usually at Asian stores, that shreds vegetables into long shoestrings.
3. Bring a pot of water to boil. Add the carrots and blanch for 10 seconds—yes, 10 seconds. Strain the carrots and rinse with cold water. Blanching softens the carrots a touch.
4. Drizzle olive oil and sauce and refrigerate for an hour to allow carrots to absorb the flavors.

The sellers make a spicy version of this salad. To add a touch of heat, mix in a little chili sauce or diced chili pepper.

Green Papaya Salad (Som Tom)

Som Tom is my absolute favorite Thai dish. We can easily find it in any food cart on any street in Thailand. Street vendors offer two versions: green papaya and mango. Thai women claim they stay skinny by eating this dish.

Street vendors tone down the spiciness of this dish when selling it to foreigners. They are surprised when I ask for regular spiciness. When eating this dish, sweat would pour from my red face. While eating, I must pause to breathe in and out to dissipate the heat blast in my mouth. Of course, I loved watching the British tourists wince and suffer as they tried to eat this spicy salad. Figure 8 shows my homemade version of Som Tom.

Figure 8. Green Papaya (Som Tom) Salad

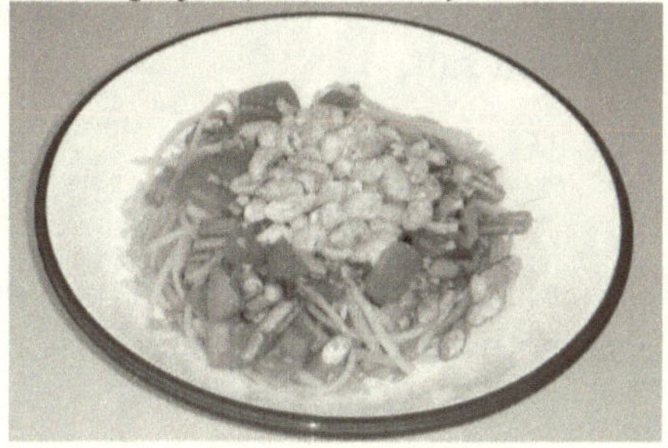

Ingredients

- 2 bowls green raw papaya, julienne
- 10 green beans, cut diagonally into small pieces
- 5 garlic cloves, finely diced
- 4 Roma or cherry tomatoes, chopped in half and sliced
- 6 red, small chili peppers (spicy)
- 2 tablespoons palm sugar, or 1 tablespoon table sugar
- 1/4 cup freshly squeezed lime juice
- 1/2 cup Thai fish sauce
- 1/2 cup unsalted peanuts, roasted
- 1/2 cup dried, miniature prawns (optional)
- 1 small raw crab (optional)

Directions

1. Ripe papaya has yellow skin and orange flesh. Meanwhile, green papaya has a green skin with light green (or pinkish) flesh. I prefer Julienne the green papaya for thick shoestrings similar to linguine.
2. I mix the garlic, chilies, sugar, lime juice, and Thai fish sauce together and let it sit for a while to absorb all the flavors. The street vendors always use a mortar and pestle to blend and mash the ingredients.
3. Mix the remaining ingredients and add the sauce.
4. American peanuts are salty. To re-roast, rinse the salty peanuts in water to remove the salt and bake on a cookie sheet for 10 minutes at 300 ^{0}F (or 150 ^{0}C). Thai fish sauce contains plenty of salt, so adding salty peanuts adds too much salt.

Notes:

- Thai fish sauce is a hallmark of Thai cooking. Producers age the sauce by fermenting anchovies in brine.

- I always ask to omit the raw crab. Otherwise, we are asking for trouble with raw seafood stored on a street cart all day in tropical temperatures.
- I can never find the dried, miniature prawns in Malaysian stores and omit this ingredient too.

Homemade Salsa

Once we taste homemade salsa, we can never return to the jar. I add fresh salsa on top of omelets, Mexican food, or just a dip for my tortilla chips, which Figure 9 shows.

Figure 9. Homemade Salsa

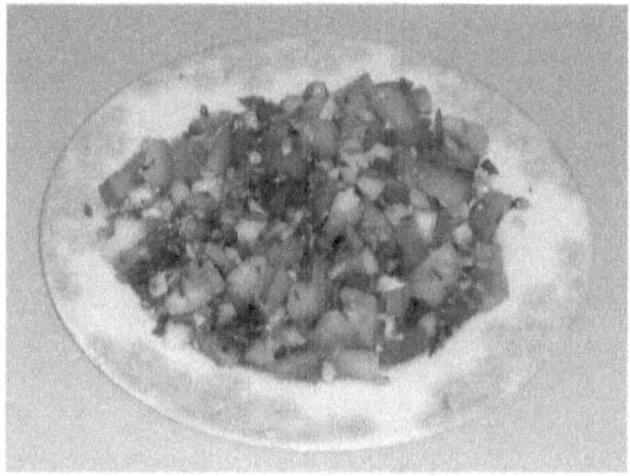

Ingredients
- 5 red tomatoes, diced
- 1 red or yellow onion, diced
- 2 green onions, diced
- 8 cloves garlic, finely diced
- 4 limes, freshly squeezed lime juice, or 2 tablespoons vinegar
- 4 jalapeno peppers, finely diced
- 1 teaspoon red chili powder
- 1/2 teaspoon cumin
- 1 teaspoon salt
- 1 teaspoon black pepper
- 1/4 cup minced cilantro (optional)

Directions

1. Mix all ingredients. Refrigerate. We cannot get more straightforward than that. In some recipes, simmer the sauce over low heat. However, I want raw and uncooked vegetables and seasonings to maintain the vitamins and minerals.

Note: Fresh pineapple or mango chunks go well with salsa.

Lime Juice

In Malaysia, many cafes and restaurants offer fresh lime juice. I drink lime juice on a regular basis, as Figure 10 depicts. It serves as an excellent mixer for tequila and whiskey.

Figure 10. Lime Juice

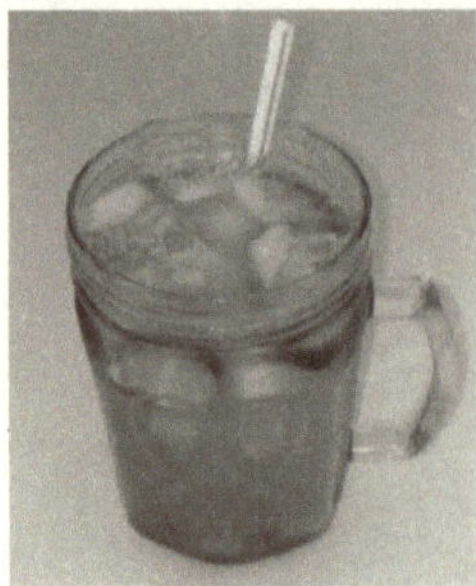

Ingredients
- 5 tablespoons sugar
- 5 cups water
- 10 small limes
- Ice

Directions

1. Slice limes in half. Place all ingredients in a bowl or container. Add 5 cups boiling water. The hot water also removes some of the oils from the skin.

2. Allow the mixture to cool, then pass it through a wire mesh to remove all the limes and seeds. I also squeeze the limes to extract all the juice.
3. Pour into a glass filled with ice. Garnish with lime halves. Refrigerate the remainder.
4. I started substituting stevia for sugar. Although I do not follow the keto diet strictly, I look for ways to decrease my sugar and starch intake.

Lime Soda

Pharmacies sold sodas as health tonics and energy drinks in the late 19th century. For example, Dr Pepper, the first soda, was invented as an energy drink and brain tonic [301]. Meanwhile, the original 7-up contained a mood stabilizer called lithium citrate [301]. Then everyone drank Coca-Cola to rejuvenate their health, strength, and vitality [301].

Thus, I resurrect soda's original purpose as a health drink using 100% natural juices, as shown in Figure 11.

Figure 11. Lime Soda

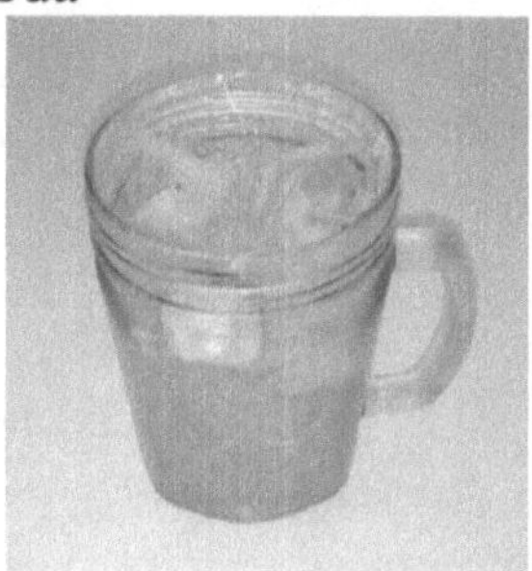

Ingredients
- 1 cup sugar
- 1 cup water
- 1 tablespoon fresh lime zest
- 2/3 cup freshly squeezed lime juice
- Carbonated water
- Ice

Directions

1. If the grater makes slivers, use it to get a tablespoon of lime zest. If the zest is a fine powder, reduce it to a teaspoon.
2. Add zest, water, and sugar to a saucepan and stir over low heat. Once all the sugar dissolves, remove the heat and allow it to cool.
3. Add the freshly squeezed lime juice and refrigerate. Also, chill the carbonated water. The coldness keeps the carbon dioxide dissolved in the water.
4. Add 1/3 syrup and 2/3 carbonated water to make the soda, mix, and add ice.

We can adjust the recipe for other flavors.

Lemon soda
- Replace the lime zest with lemon zest.
- Replace lime juice with freshly squeezed lemon juice.

Orange soda
- Replace the lime zest with orange zest.
- Replace lime juice with freshly squeezed orange juice.

Cream soda
- Replace the lime zest with a tablespoon of vanilla.
- Add two tablespoons of fresh lemon or lime juice. The name of the cream soda may come from cream of tartar, another sour agent used in cream soda.
- Please do not mix dairy cream with soda since the cream is alkaline, and carbonated water is slightly acidic. Acid causes the milk fat to separate unless one wants cottage cheese in their soda.

Note: My friends and I were surprised by the deliciousness of these homemade sodas.

Soursop (Guyabano) Smoothie

I fell in love with the soursop smoothie when I first tried it in Brunei at the mall. Some people eat soursop for its health and anti-cancer properties. However, no scientific evidence supports the power of soursop to combat cancer. Figure 12 shows a picture of a soursop with the soursop smoothie to the right. Please distinguish soursop from durian. Durian, another Asian favorite fruit, emits a strong, reeking, dead-body smell. Trust me, I can smell the foul-smelling durian a block away. It is impossible to confuse a soursop and a durian.

Figure 12. Soursop (or Guyabano) Smoothie

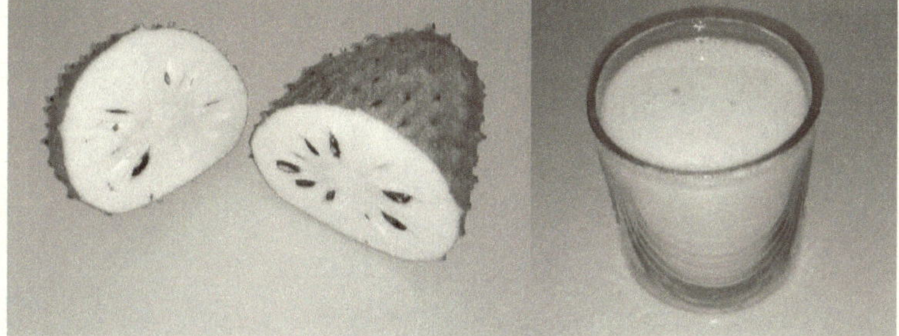

Ingredients
- 3 chunks Soursop
- 1 cup vanilla or plain yogurt
- Honey
- Ice cubes

Directions
1. Slice the Soursop in half and carefully peel the skin with a knife. Slice flesh into small one-inch (or 2.5 cm) cubes. We must remove the seeds from the cubes and cut them small.
2. Add yogurt, a cup of Soursop chunks, and several ice cubes. Drizzle a little honey and blend. Add additional

honey and ice to get the desired sweetness and consistency.

We freeze the leftover Soursop if we use it for future smoothies.

Three Sour

I discovered Three Sour in the Chinese cafes in Malaysia, and it has become one of my favorite drinks. Three Sour comes from lemon, lime, and sour plum and is shown in Figure 13.

One of the things I love about Three Sour is its versatility. On my fasting days, I enjoy a modified version, omitting the sugar and adding a ½ teaspoon of Himalayan salt for a unique twist. This adaptability allows us to tailor the recipe to our preferences and dietary needs.

Figure 13. Three Sour

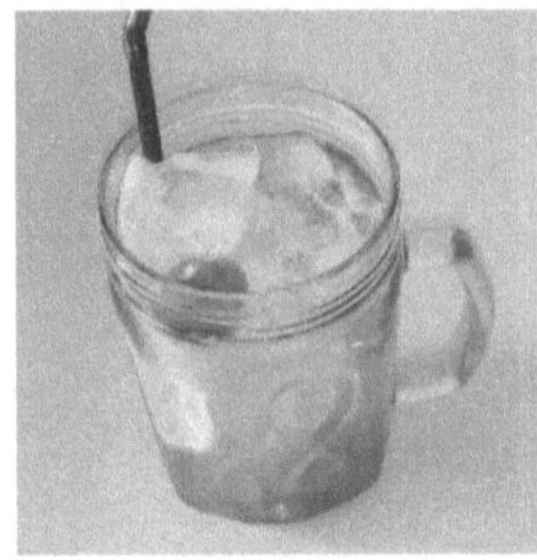

Ingredients
- 10 small limes
- 10 lemon slices
- 5 sour or salty plums
- 5 tablespoons table sugar or sugar substitute
- 5 cups boiling water
- Ice

Directions

1. Slice limes in half and place all ingredients into a container or bowl.
2. Add boiling water, stir to dissolve the sugar, and allow the mixture to cool.
3. Strain the mixture through a wire mesh to remove the seeds. I also squeeze all the juice from the limes and lemons.
4. Pour into a glass with ice. Add freshly sliced lime and lemon and one plum as a garnish.

I prefer the dried sour plum, but Asian stores sell sour plums in brine. Although the salty plum is a good choice, the salt neutralizes the sourness of the drink.

11. The Conclusion

"Fifty is the new thirty, via intermittent fasting."

– Ken Szulczyk

I added my quote to express the quintessential impact of fasting on my life. I am in better shape at 54 than I was at 30. Heck, I am in better shape than when I was 20.

When I started fasting, I did not think much about it except I would benefit from autophagy. However, the weight melted off my body, while my waist size shrank from a 38 to a 33 with little effort. The 33-waist has even become loose. I could not squeeze into a 33-inch waist since high school. Thus, I knew fasting held something special. Come on; we all know. The greatest prophets, Jesus, Muhammad, and Buddha all fasted. So, fasting was never secret knowledge. I read the Bible several times and skipped the fasting passages without thought or interest. I heard someone mention intermittent fasting, and it piqued my curiosity. Then I watched the YouTube videos.

After starting intermittent fasting, I witnessed performance improvements in the gym. I exercised with heavier weights and greater repetitions. Then I started running 6.21 miles (or 10 km) nonstop. I could not run that distance nonstop as a young man. Fasting has transformed me into an athlete.

In the past, I researched many herbs and supplements, searching for the fountain of youth in a bottle. Out of all the medicines, medical technology, and herbs that we have access to, fasting blows all other alternatives out of the water. Nothing comes a close second. Do not get me wrong. Exercise, diet restriction, and several supplements are great for the body, but they do not compete with fasting. Fasting switches on the body's repair mechanisms via autophagy, removal or regeneration of the senescent cells, and activating the longevity genes.

After fasting for four years, fasting has become easy. Also, I no longer get the white, coated tongue, and the euphoria has weakened considerably. I often feel no difference between fasting and feasting, even though I have not eaten for 30 hours or more. Thus, I ask myself several questions.

Am I abusing intermittent fasting? Am I fasting too frequently, causing fasting to lose its effectiveness? A good research question is whether the power of fasting weakens each time we use it. Another question related to fasting is the long-term effects on the body. I do not know the answer to these questions. However, exercise and calorie restriction place stress on the body. The lungs, heart, and blood transport oxygen more efficiently to the body during aerobic exercise, while anaerobic exercise strengthens the muscles and bones. Then the body lowers metabolism for calorie restriction to conserve energy. Therefore, as an ingenious machine, the body ensures survival in stressful environments. Thus, the body adapts to stress.

We know fasting places more stress on the body than exercise and calorie restriction. Hence, the body adapts and tries to minimize this stress. For example, Dr. Shelton noticed patients lost less weight on second and third fasts because the body conserves its resources efficiently [3]. Animal studies also highlight the impact of fasting. The fasted mice gained 10% more body weight than the control group [104, 199], while another study on fasted rabbits showed a 50% gain in weight [14]. Therefore, the mice's and rabbits' bodies had adapted to the stress of fasting, or their digestive system processed food more efficiently [14].

Another question I have is, do our bodies become more efficient in entering the fasting state each time we fast? Then autophagy and the repair processes become more efficient. Or must we fast for longer and longer periods to attain the same benefits of fasting? Unfortunately, the research has just started to unravel the mysteries of fasting.

I have another question. Will fasting extend my lifespan? I think I have to say yes because old age started to catch up with me at 50 as I suffered from chronic allergies, recurring infections and colds, and constant digestive issues with persistent diarrhea. I gobbled down the antihistamines and Imodium three or more times per week. My knee joints were stiff, and I started to put on the weight. I was in the worst shape of my life. Occasionally, I would get these chest pains as if someone were stabbing at my chest with an ice-cold ice pick.

Then I tried intermittent fasting. Poof! All my ailments have disappeared. The weight melted off; my BMI dropped 4%, and the joint stiffness disappeared. I do not get chest pains anymore. If I can delay the effects of aging another 20 years, I will have no problem reaching 100 years old. Fasting gives us the means to age gracefully like a fine wine. We get better with age. Unfortunately, we will not live to the same age as Adam, over 900 years old. We need an act of God or some magic concoction to live that long.

My last question is whether the efficacy of fasting depends on age. For example, if a 25-year-old, 50-year-old, and 75-year-old fasted for 24 hours, is the fasting process identical for all people? When we age, our hormone levels decline, while our cells fill with garbage. Our bodies brim with senescent zombie cells. Do fasting repair processes also become less efficient over time? We would expect the 75-year-old to need more bouts of fasting since he or she is more likely to have health problems, but does the aging process also reduce the effectiveness of fasting? Unfortunately, we already know the answer to this one. Several studies indicate that autophagy weakens as we age [42]. We should fast for longer durations and more frequently to offset weakening autophagy. However, my landlord in Las Vegas showed improvement in health at 85. That gives me hope.

I hope the readers have enjoyed this book. If we must take away one thing, we use fasting to enjoy life and keep our bodies healthy. We have been on this planet for a short time. We are all passengers on a bullet train as we watch the scenes of life fly by the window. We can use intermittent fasting to make the train ride more enjoyable and delay the final destination a little longer.

Let us make the planet a better place while living life to the fullest. By utilizing the power of fasting, we can all age gracefully.

12. References

[1]   Sinclair, U. 1911 *The Fasting Cure*: Chet Day's Health and Beyond Online

[2]   Dewey, E.H. 1900 *The No Breakfast Plan and the Fasting-Cure* Project Gutenberg: Edward Hooker Dewey

[3]   Shelton, H.M. 1978 *The Science and Fine Art of Fasting* 5th ed: Dr. Shelton's Health School

[4]   U.S. Geological Survey. *The Water in You*. 2018; Available from: https://water.usgs.gov/edu/propertyyou.html.

[5]   The New King James Version *The Holy Bible*

[6]   Cadotte, G.K. 2022 *Using Meditation to Tune Consciousness* Udemy

[7]   Laidlaw, J. 2005 A Life Worth Leaving: Fasting to Death as Telos of a Jain Religious Life *Economy and Society* 34(2): pp 178-199

[8]   Buddha Dharma Education Association. *A Monk's Dream Comes to Life*. 2012; Available from: https://www.buddhanet.net/e-learning/buddhistworld/wat_m5.htm.

[9]   Fuhrman, J. 1995 *Fasting and Eating for Health*: St. Martin's Press

[10]   Thompson, C. 2018 *Art of Intermittent Fasting - How to Lose Weight, Shed Fat, and Live a Healthier Life*

[11]   Fung, J. and J. Moore 2016 *The Complete Guide to Fasting: Heal Your Body through Intermittent, Alternate-Day, and Extended Fasting*: Victory Belt Publishing

[12]   Fung, J. 2016 *The Obesity Code: Unlocking the Secrets of Weight Loss*

[13]   Awad, S., et al. 2010 The Effects of Fasting and Refeeding with a 'Metabolic Preconditioning' drink on Substrate Reserves and Mononuclear Cell Mitochondrial Function *Clinical Nutrition* 29(4): pp 538-544

[14]   Devries, A. 1963 *Therapeutic Fasting*: Chandler Book Co.

[15]   Pet MD. *Fatty Liver Disease in Cats*. 2018; Available from: https://www.petmd.com/cat/conditions/digestive/c_ct_hepatic_lipidosis

[16]   Kolb, H., et al. 2021 Ketone Bodies: From Enemy to Friend and Guardian Angel *BMC Medicine* 19(1): pp 1-15

[17]   Kerndt, P.R., et al. 1982 Fasting: The History, Pathophysiology and Complications *Western Journal of Medicine* 137(5): pp 379

[18]   Veech, R.L., et al. 2001 Ketone Bodies, Potential Therapeutic Uses *IUBMB Life* 51(4): pp 241-247

[19]   Owen, O.E., et al. 1969 Liver and Kidney Metabolism During Prolonged Starvation *The Journal of Clinical Investigation* 48(3): pp 574-583

[20]   Johnson, J.B., et al. 2007 Alternate Day Calorie Restriction Improves Clinical Findings and Reduces Markers of Oxidative Stress and Inflammation in Overweight Adults with Moderate Asthma *Free Radical Biology and Medicine* 42(5): pp 665-674

[21]   Duncan, G.G. 1963 Intermittent Fasts in the Correction and Control of Intractable Obesity *Transactions of the American Clinical and Climatological Association* 74: pp 121

[22]   Bak, A.M., et al. 2018 Prolonged Fasting-Induced Metabolic Signatures in Human Skeletal Muscle of Lean and Obese Men *PloS One* 13(9): pp e0200817

[23]   Zauner, C., et al. 2000 Resting Energy Expenditure in Short-Term Starvation Is Increased as a Result of an Increase in Serum Norepinephrine *The American Journal of Clinical Nutrition* 71(6): pp 1511-1515

[24]   Crook, M., V. Hally, and J. Panteli 2001 The Importance of the Refeeding Syndrome *Nutrition* 17(7-8): pp 632-637

[25]   Biden, T.J. and K.W. Taylor 1983 Effects of Ketone Bodies on Insulin Release and Islet-Cell Metabolism in the Rat *Biochemical Journal* 212(2): pp 371-377

[26]   Madison, L.L., et al. 1964 The Hypoglycemic Action of Ketones. Ii. Evidence for a Stimulatory Feedback of Ketones on the Pancreatic Beta Cells *The Journal of Clinical Investigation* 43(3): pp 408-415

[27]   Musa-Veloso, K., S.S. Likhodii, and S.C. Cunnane 2002 Breath Acetone Is a Reliable Indicator of Ketosis in Adults Consuming Ketogenic Meals *The American journal of Clinical Nutrition* 76(1): pp 65-70

[28]   Cott, A. 1971 Controlled Fasting Treatment of Schizophrenia in Ussr *Schizophrenia* 3(1): pp 2-10

[29]   Moser, I. 1997 *How and When to Be Your Own Doctor*: Prabhat Prakashan

[30]   Heilbronn, L.K., et al. 2005 Glucose Tolerance and Skeletal Muscle Gene Expression in Response to Alternate Day Fasting *Obesity Research* 13(3): pp 574-581

[31]   de Toledo, F.W., et al. 2019 Safety, Health Improvement and Well-Being During a 4 to 21-Day Fasting Period in an Observational Study Including 1422 Subjects *PloS One* 14(1): pp 1-23

[32]   Arai, Y., et al. 2015 Inflammation, but Not Telomere Length, Predicts Successful Ageing at Extreme Old Age: A Longitudinal Study of Semi-Supercentenarians *EBioMedicine* 2(10): pp 1549-1558

[33]   Almeneessier, A.S., et al. 2019 The Effects of Diurnal Intermittent Fasting on Proinflammatory Cytokine Levels While Controlling for Sleep/Wake Pattern, Meal Composition and Energy Expenditure *PLoS One* 14(12): pp e0226034

[34]   Fuhrman, J. and B. Sarter 2002 Brief Case Reports of Medically Supervised, Water-Only Fasting Associated with Remission of Autoimmune Disease *Alternative Therapies in Health and Medicine*

[35]   Buhner, S.H. *The Health Benefits of Water Fasting*. 2003; Available from: www.gaianstudies.org/articles4.htm.

[36]   Choi, I.Y., C. Lee, and V.D. Longo 2017 Nutrition and Fasting Mimicking Diets in the Prevention and Treatment of Autoimmune

Diseases and Immunosenescence *Molecular and Cellular Endocrinology* 455: pp 4-12

[37] Longo, V.D. and M.P. Mattson 2014 Fasting: Molecular Mechanisms and Clinical Applications *Cell Metabolism* 19(2): pp 181-192

[38] Sisson, M. 2011 *The Myriad Benefits of Intermittent Fasting* Mark's Daily Apple

[39] Nakamura, S., et al. 2019 Suppression of Autophagic Activity by Rubicon Is a Signature of Aging *Nature Communications* 10(1): pp 847

[40] Sachdeva, U.M. and C.B. Thompson 2008 Diurnal Rhythms of Autophagy: Implications for Cell Biology and Human Disease *Autophagy* 4(5): pp 581-589

[41] Rubinsztein, D.C., G. Mariño, and G. Kroemer 2011 Autophagy and Aging *Cell* 146(5): pp 682-695

[42] Koutouroushis, C. and O. Sarkar 2021 Role of Autophagy in Cardiovascular Disease and Aging *Cureus* 13(11)

[43] Hippert, M.M., P.S. O'Toole, and A. Thorburn 2006 Autophagy in Cancer: Good, Bad, or Both? *Cancer Research* 66(19): pp 9349-9351

[44] Vicencio, J.M., et al. 2008 Senescence, Apoptosis or Autophagy? *Gerontology* 54(2): pp 92-99

[45] Vellai, T., et al. 2009 The Regulation of Aging: Does Autophagy Underlie Longevity? *Trends in Cell Biology* 19(10): pp 487-494

[46] Ouimet, M., et al. 2011 Autophagy Regulates Cholesterol Efflux from Macrophage Foam Cells Via Lysosomal Acid Lipase *Cell Metabolism* 13(6): pp 655-667

[47] Hay, N. and N. Sonenberg 2004 Upstream and Downstream of Mtor *Genes and Development* 18: pp 1926-1945

[48] Wilhelmi de Toledo, F., et al. 2020 Unravelling the Health Effects of Fasting: A Long Road from Obesity Treatment to Healthy Life Span Increase and Improved Cognition *Annals of Medicine* 52(5): pp 147-161

[49] Heilbronn, L.K., et al. 2005 Alternate-Day Fasting in Nonobese Subjects: Effects on Body Weight, Body Composition, and Energy Metabolism *The American Journal of Clinical Nutrition* 81(1): pp 69-73

[50] Malinowski, B., et al. 2019 Intermittent Fasting in Cardiovascular Disorders—an Overview *Nutrients* 11(3): pp 673

[51] Wilhelmi de Toledo, F., et al. 2020 Influence of Long-Term Fasting on Blood Redox Status in Humans *Antioxidants* 9(6): pp 496

[52] McDaniel, S.S., et al. 2011 The Ketogenic Diet Inhibits the Mammalian Target of Rapamycin (Mtor) Pathway *Epilepsia* 52(3): pp e7-e11

[53] Zyrowski, N. *Best Hours for Intermittent Fasting | the Golden Hours.* 2018; Available from: https://www.youtube.com/watch?v=MxrNxxd3gMI.

[54] Jamshed, H., et al. 2019 Early Time-Restricted Feeding Improves 24-Hour Glucose Levels and Affects Markers of the Circadian Clock, Aging, and Autophagy in Humans *Nutrients* 11(6): pp 1234

[55]   Yoshii, S.R. and N. Mizushima 2017 Monitoring and Measuring Autophagy *International Journal of Molecular Sciences* 18(9): pp 1865

[56]   Land, S. 2019 *Metabolic Autophagy: Practice Intermittent Fasting and Resistance Training to Build Muscle and Promote Longevity (Metabolic Autophagy Diet Book 1)* Amazon Digital Services LLC

[57]   Williamson, D.L., et al. 2006 Exercise-Induced Alterations in Extracellular Signal-Regulated Kinase 1/2 and Mammalian Target of Rapamycin (Mtor) Signalling to Regulatory Mechanisms of Mrna Translation in Mouse Muscle *The Journal of Physiology* 573(2): pp 497-510

[58]   Vindis, C. 2015 Autophagy: An Emerging Therapeutic Target in Vascular Diseases *British Journal of Pharmacology* 172(9): pp 2167-2178

[59]   Pietrocola, F., et al. 2014 Coffee Induces Autophagy in Vivo *Cell Cycle* 13(12): pp 1987-1994

[60]   Gump, J.M. and A. Thorburn 2011 Autophagy and Apoptosis: What Is the Connection? *Trends in Cell Biology* 21(7): pp 387-392

[61]   Klionsky, D.J., A.M. Cuervo, and P.O. Seglen 2007 Methods for Monitoring Autophagy from Yeast to Human *Autophagy* 3(3): pp 181-206

[62]   Alirezaei, M., et al. 2010 Short-Term Fasting Induces Profound Neuronal Autophagy *Autophagy* 6(6): pp 702-710

[63]   Gannon, A.M., M.R. Stämpfli, and W.G. Foster 2013 Cigarette Smoke Exposure Elicits Increased Autophagy and Dysregulation of Mitochondrial Dynamics in Murine Granulosa Cells *Biology of Reproduction* 88(3): pp 63, 1-11

[64]   Finn, P.F. and J.F. Dice 2005 Ketone Bodies Stimulate Chaperone-Mediated Autophagy *Journal of Biological Chemistry* 280(27): pp 25864-25870

[65]   McCarty, M.F., J.J. DiNicolantonio, and J.H. O'Keefe 2015 Ketosis May Promote Brain Macroautophagy by Activating Sirt1 and Hypoxia-Inducible Factor-1 *Medical Hypotheses* 85(5): pp 631-639

[66]   Newman, J.C. and E. Verdin 2014 Ketone Bodies as Signaling Metabolites *Trends in Endocrinology & Metabolism* 25(1): pp 42-52

[67]   Zhou, J., et al. 2014 Epigallocatechin-3-Gallate (Egcg), a Green Tea Polyphenol, Stimulates Hepatic Autophagy and Lipid Clearance *PloS One* 9(1): pp e87161

[68]   Nunes, P., et al. 2013 Hypertonic Stress Promotes Autophagy and Microtubule-Dependent Autophagosomal Clusters *Autophagy* 9(4): pp 550-567

[69]   Ros, M. and J.M. Carrascosa 2020 Current Nutritional and Pharmacological Anti-Aging Interventions *Biochimica et Biophysica Acta (BBA)-Molecular Basis of Disease* 1866(3): pp 165612

[70] Wang, A., et al. 2016 Opposing Effects of Fasting Metabolism on Tissue Tolerance in Bacterial and Viral Inflammation *Cell* 166(6): pp 1512-1525. e12

[71] Ealey, K.N., J. Phillips, and H.-K. Sung 2021 Covid-19 and Obesity: Fighting Two Pandemics with Intermittent Fasting *Trends in Endocrinology & Metabolism* 32(9): pp 706-720

[72] Remuzzi, A. and G. Remuzzi 2020 Covid-19 and Italy: What Next? *The Lancet* 395(10231): pp 1225-1228

[73] Wu, Z. and J.M. McGoogan 2020 Characteristics of and Important Lessons from the Coronavirus Disease 2019 (Covid-19) Outbreak in China: Summary of a Report of 72 314 Cases from the Chinese Center for Disease Control and Prevention *JAMA* 323(13): pp 1239-1242

[74] Zheng, Y.-Y., et al. 2020 Covid-19 and the Cardiovascular System *Nature Reviews Cardiology* 17(5): pp 259-260

[75] Covid, C., et al. 2020 *Severe Outcomes among Patients with Coronavirus Disease 2019 (Covid-19)—United States, February 12– March 16, 2020* in *Morbidity and Mortality Weekly Report* pp 343

[76] Guan, W.-j., et al. 2020 Clinical Characteristics of Coronavirus Disease 2019 in China *New England Journal of Medicine* 382(18): pp 1708-1720

[77] Mo'ez, A.-I.E., et al. 2020 Ramadan Intermittent Fasting and Immunity: An Important Topic in the Era of Covid-19 *Annals of Thoracic Medicine* 15(3): pp 125

[78] Hannan, M.A., et al. 2020 Intermittent Fasting, a Possible Priming Tool for Host Defense against Sars-Cov-2 Infection: Crosstalk among Calorie Restriction, Autophagy and Immune Response *Immunology Letters* 226: pp 38-45

[79] Alahmad, B., et al. 2020 Fasting Blood Glucose and Covid-19 Severity: Nonlinearity Matters *Diabetes Care* 43(12): pp 3113-3116

[80] Wang, W., et al. 2011 Fasting Plasma Glucose Is an Independent Predictor for Severity of H1n1 Pneumonia *BMC Infectious Diseases* 11(1): pp 1-6

[81] Mccalmon, S., et al. 2021 Fasting Off "the Covid-19" *Missouri Medicine* 118(2): pp 164

[82] Martin, B., M.P. Mattson, and S. Maudsley 2006 Caloric Restriction and Intermittent Fasting: Two Potential Diets for Successful Brain Aging *Ageing Research Reviews* 5(3): pp 332-353

[83] Duan, W., Z. Guo, and M.P. Mattson 2001 Brain-Derived Neurotrophic Factor Mediates an Excitoprotective Effect of Dietary Restriction in Mice *Journal of Neurochemistry* 76(2): pp 619-626

[84] Patterson, R.E. and D.D. Sears 2017 Metabolic Effects of Intermittent Fasting *Annual Review of Nutrition* 37

[85] Nilsson, P., et al. 2013 Aβ Secretion and Plaque Formation Depend on Autophagy *Cell Reports* 5(1): pp 61-69

[86] Halagappa, V.K.M., et al. 2007 Intermittent Fasting and Caloric Restriction Ameliorate Age-Related Behavioral Deficits in the Triple-

Transgenic Mouse Model of Alzheimer's Disease *Neurobiology of Disease* 26(1): pp 212-220

[87]   Hoeffer, C.A. and E. Klann 2010 Mtor Signaling: At the Crossroads of Plasticity, Memory and Disease *Trends in Neurosciences* 33(2): pp 67-75

[88]   Li, L., Z. Wang, and Z. Zuo 2013 Chronic Intermittent Fasting Improves Cognitive Functions and Brain Structures in Mice *PloS One* 8(6): pp e66069

[89]   Mattson, M.P. 2005 Energy Intake, Meal Frequency, and Health: A Neurobiological Perspective *Annual Review of Nutrition* 25: pp 237-260

[90]   Arumugam, T.V., et al. 2010 Age and Energy Intake Interact to Modify Cell Stress Pathways and Stroke Outcome *Annals of Neurology* 67(1): pp 41-52

[91]   Duan, W., et al. 2003 Dietary Restriction Normalizes Glucose Metabolism and Bdnf Levels, Slows Disease Progression, and Increases Survival in Huntingtin Mutant Mice *Proceedings of the National Academy of Sciences* 100(5): pp 2911-2916

[92]   Lee, J., et al. 2000 Dietary Restriction Increases the Number of Newly Generated Neural Cells, and Induces Bdnf Expression, in the Dentate Gyrus of Rats *Journal of Molecular Neuroscience* 15(2): pp 99-108

[93]   Jeong, M.-a., et al. 2011 Intermittent Fasting Improves Functional Recovery after Rat Thoracic Contusion Spinal Cord Injury *Journal of Neurotrauma* 28(3): pp 479-492

[94]   Hunter, P. 2012 The Inflammation Theory of Disease: The Growing Realization That Chronic Inflammation Is Crucial in Many Diseases Opens New Avenues for Treatment *EMBO Reports* 13(11): pp 968-970

[95]   Trafton, A. 2016 *How Cancer Cells Fuel Their Growth*. MIT News,

[96]   Gallagher, E.J. and D. LeRoith 2011 Minireview: Igf, Insulin, and Cancer *Endocrinology* 152(7): pp 2546-2551

[97]   Varady, K.A., D. Roohk, and M.K. Hellerstein 2007 Dose Effects of Modified Alternate-Day Fasting Regimens on in Vivo Cell Proliferation and Plasma Insulin-Like Growth Factor-1 in Mice *Journal of Applied Physiology* 103(2): pp 547-551

[98]   Bianchini, F., R. Kaaks, and H. Vainio 2002 Overweight, Obesity, and Cancer Risk *The Lancet Oncology* 3(9): pp 565-574

[99]   Nencioni, A., et al. 2018 Fasting and Cancer: Molecular Mechanisms and Clinical Application *Nature Reviews Cancer* 18(11): pp 707-719

[100]   Cheng, C.-W., et al. 2014 Prolonged Fasting Reduces Igf-1/Pka to Promote Hematopoietic-Stem-Cell-Based Regeneration and Reverse Immunosuppression *Cell Stem Cell* 14(6): pp 810-823

[101]   Ravichandran, M., G. Grandl, and M. Ristow 2017 Dietary Carbohydrates Impair Healthspan and Promote Mortality *Cell Metabolism* 26(4): pp 585-587

[102] Rocha, N.S., et al. 2002 Effects of Fasting and Intermittent Fasting on Rat Hepatocarcinogenesis Induced by Diethylnitrosamine *Teratogenesis, Carcinogenesis, and Mutagenesis* 22(2): pp 129-138

[103] Lee, C., et al. 2012 Fasting Cycles Retard Growth of Tumors and Sensitize a Range of Cancer Cell Types to Chemotherapy *Science Translational Medicine* 4(124): pp 124ra27-124ra27

[104] Descamps, O., et al. 2005 Mitochondrial Production of Reactive Oxygen Species and Incidence of Age-Associated Lymphoma in Of1 Mice: Effect of Alternate-Day Fasting *Mechanisms of Ageing and Development* 126(11): pp 1185-1191

[105] Rahbar, A.R., et al. 2019 Effects of Intermittent Fasting During Ramadan on Insulin-Like Growth Factor-1, Interleukin 2, and Lipid Profile in Healthy Muslims *International Journal of Preventive Medicine* 10

[106] Jiang, Y., et al. 2021 Five-Day Water-Only Fasting Decreased Metabolic-Syndrome Risk Factors and Increased Anti-Aging Biomarkers without Toxicity in a Clinical Trial of Normal-Weight Individuals *Clinical and Translational Medicine* 11(8): pp e502

[107] Anson, R.M., et al. 2003 Intermittent Fasting Dissociates Beneficial Effects of Dietary Restriction on Glucose Metabolism and Neuronal Resistance to Injury from Calorie Intake *Proceedings of the National Academy of Sciences* 100(10): pp 6216-6220

[108] Wan, R., S. Camandola, and M.P. Mattson 2003 Intermittent Fasting and Dietary Supplementation with 2-Deoxy-D-Glucose Improve Functional and Metabolic Cardiovascular Risk Factors in Rats *The FASEB Journal* 17(9): pp 1133-1134

[109] Longo, V.D., et al. 2015 Interventions to Slow Aging in Humans: Are We Ready? *Aging Cell* 14(4): pp 497-510

[110] Raffaghello, L., et al. 2008 Starvation-Dependent Differential Stress Resistance Protects Normal but Not Cancer Cells against High-Dose Chemotherapy *Proceedings of the National Academy of Sciences* 105(24): pp 8215-8220

[111] Hu, Y.-L., et al. 2012 Hypoxia-Induced Autophagy Promotes Tumor Cell Survival and Adaptation to Antiangiogenic Treatment in Glioblastoma *Cancer Research* 72(7): pp 1773-1783

[112] Kenific, C.M., A. Thorburn, and J. Debnath 2010 Autophagy and Metastasis: Another Double-Edged Sword *Current Opinion in Cell Biology* 22(2): pp 241-245

[113] Thomas II, J., et al. 2010 Effect of Intermittent Fasting on Prostate Cancer Tumor Growth in a Mouse Model *Prostate Cancer and Prostatic Diseases* 13(4): pp 350

[114] Mayo Clinic. *Stem Cells: What They Are and What They Do.* 2018; Available from: https://www.mayoclinic.org/tests-procedures/bone-marrow-transplant/in-depth/stem-cells/art-20048117.

[115]   Ho, A.D., W. Wagner, and U. Mahlknecht 2005 Stem Cells and Ageing: The Potential of Stem Cells to Overcome Age-Related Deteriorations of the Body in Regenerative Medicine *EMBO Reports* 6(S1): pp S35-S38

[116]   Jarreau, P.B. *Eating (or Rather, Fasting) Our Way to Rejuvenated Stem Cells?* 2018; Available from: https://medium.com/lifeomic/eating-or-rather-fasting-our-way-to-rejuvenated-stem-cells-e4302a49e597.

[117]   Mihaylova, M.M., et al. 2018 Fasting Activates Fatty Acid Oxidation to Enhance Intestinal Stem Cell Function During Homeostasis and Aging *Cell Stem Cell* 22(5): pp 769-778

[118]   Godínez-Victoria, M., et al. 2014 Intermittent Fasting Promotes Bacterial Clearance and Intestinal I G a Production in Salmonella Typhimurium-Infected Mice *Scandinavian Journal of Immunology* 79(5): pp 315-324

[119]   Varady, K.A., et al. 2009 Short-Term Modified Alternate-Day Fasting: A Novel Dietary Strategy for Weight Loss and Cardioprotection in Obese Adults *The American Journal of Clinical Nutrition* 90(5): pp 1138-1143

[120]   Gabel, K., et al. 2018 Effects of 8-Hour Time Restricted Feeding on Body Weight and Metabolic Disease Risk Factors in Obese Adults: A Pilot Study *Nutrition and Healthy Aging* 4(4): pp 345-353

[121]   Luo, E.K. *Everything You Need to Know About High Cholesterol.* 2018; Available from: https://www.healthline.com/health/high-cholesterol.

[122]   Ahmet, I., et al. 2005 Cardioprotection by Intermittent Fasting in Rats *Circulation* 112(20): pp 3115-21

[123]   Wan, R., et al. 2010 Cardioprotective Effect of Intermittent Fasting Is Associated with an Elevation of Adiponectin Levels in Rats *The Journal of Nutritional Biochemistry* 21(5): pp 413-417

[124]   Bhutani, S., et al. 2010 Improvements in Coronary Heart Disease Risk Indicators by Alternate-Day Fasting Involve Adipose Tissue Modulations *Obesity* 18(11): pp 2152-2159

[125]   Tinsley, G.M. and P.M. La Bounty 2015 Effects of Intermittent Fasting on Body Composition and Clinical Health Markers in Humans *Nutrition Reviews* 73(10): pp 661-674

[126]   Hutchison, A.T., et al. 2019 Effects of Intermittent Versus Continuous Energy Intakes on Insulin Sensitivity and Metabolic Risk in Women with Overweight *Obesity* 27(1): pp 50-58

[127]   Li, A.C. and C.K. Glass 2002 The Macrophage Foam Cell as a Target for Therapeutic Intervention *Nature Medicine* 8(11): pp 1235-1242

[128]   Ye, J. and J.N. Keller 2010 Regulation of Energy Metabolism by Inflammation: A Feedback Response in Obesity and Calorie Restriction *Aging* 2(6): pp 361

[129]   Gandhi, H., A. Upaganlawar, and R. Balaraman 2010 Adipocytokines: The Pied Pipers *Journal of Pharmacology & Pharmacotherapeutics* 1(1): pp 9

[130]   Hein, D. *Coq10 and Statins: What You Need to Know.* 2016; Available from: https://www.healthline.com/health/coq10-and-statins.

[131]   Ames, B.N., et al. 1981 Uric Acid Provides an Antioxidant Defense in Humans against Oxidant-and Radical-Caused Aging and Cancer: A Hypothesis *Proceedings of the National Academy of Sciences* 78(11): pp 6858-6862

[132]   Arnason, T.G., M.W. Bowen, and K.D. Mansell 2017 Effects of Intermittent Fasting on Health Markers in Those with Type 2 Diabetes: A Pilot Study *World Journal of Diabetes* 8(4): pp 154

[133]   Carstensen, B., et al. 2016 Cancer Incidence in Persons with Type 1 Diabetes: A Five-Country Study of 9,000 Cancers in Type 1 Diabetic Individuals *Diabetologia* 59(5): pp 980-988

[134]   Allen, F.M. 1915 Prolonged Fasting in Diabetes *Journal of Experimental Medicine*

[135]   Mazur, A. 2011 Why Were "Starvation Diets" Promoted for Diabetes in the Pre-Insulin Period? *Nutrition Journal* 10(1): pp 23

[136]   Barnosky, A.R., et al. 2014 Intermittent Fasting Vs Daily Calorie Restriction for Type 2 Diabetes Prevention: A Review of Human Findings *Translational Research* 164(4): pp 302-311

[137]   Gilliland, I. 1968 Total Fasting in the Treatment of Obesity *Postgraduate Medical Journal* 44(507): pp 58

[138]   Halberg, N., et al. 2005 Effect of Intermittent Fasting and Refeeding on Insulin Action in Healthy Men *Journal of Applied Physiology* 99(6): pp 2128-2136

[139]   Blagosklonny, M.V. 2019 Rapamycin for Longevity: Opinion Article *Aging* 11(19): pp 8048

[140]   Furmli, S., et al. 2018 Therapeutic Use of Intermittent Fasting for People with Type 2 Diabetes as an Alternative to Insulin *Case Reports* 2018: pp 1-5

[141]   Rasmussen, M.H. 2010 Obesity, Growth Hormone and Weight Loss *Molecular and Cellular Endocrinology* 316(2): pp 147-153

[142]   The Aesthetic Medicine and Anti-aging Clinics of Lousinana. *How Much Does Hgh Therapy Cost?* 2018; Available from: https://theantiagingclinics.com/much-hgh-therapy-cost/.

[143]   Paulson, P. 2014 *Intermittent Fasting 101: A Simple Guide to Losing Fat, Building Muscle and Becoming an Alpha Male*: Create Space

[144]   Salgin, B., et al. 2012 The Effect of Prolonged Fasting on Levels of Growth Hormone-Binding Protein and Free Growth Hormone *Growth Hormone & IGF Research* 22(2): pp 76-81

[145]   Tavares, A.B.W., et al. 2003 Effects of Growth Hormone Administration on Muscle Strength in Men over 50 Years Old *International Journal of Endocrinology*

[146]   Arias, E. 2003 *United States Life Tables* D.o.V. Statistics Editor Centers for Disease Control and Prevention

[147]   National Center for Health Statistics 2017 *Table 14. Life Expectancy at Birth and at Age 65, by Sex: Organisation for Economic Co-Operation and Development (Oecd) Countries, Selected Years 1980–2015* C.f.D.C.a. Prevention Editor

[148]   Guinness World Records. *Oldest Person Ever.* 2018; Available from: http://www.guinnessworldrecords.com/world-records/oldest-person.

[149]   Bidwell, V. *Timeline for the Life of Dr. Herbert M. Shelton.* Available from: http://www.veganvillage.org/Article-Bio-Herbert-M-Shelton.html.

[150]   Hayflick, L. 1965 The Limited in Vitro Lifetime of Human Diploid Cell Strains *Experimental Cell Research* 37(3): pp 614-636

[151]   Hayflick, L. and P.S. Moorhead 1961 The Serial Cultivation of Human Diploid Cell Strains *Experimental Cell Research* 25(3): pp 585-621

[152]   Schmucker, D.L. and H. Sanchez 2011 Liver Regeneration and Aging: A Current Perspective *Current Gerontology and Geriatrics Research* 2011

[153]   Ceolotto, G., et al. 2004 Insulin Generates Free Radicals by an Nad (P) H, Phosphatidylinositol 3′-Kinase-Dependent Mechanism in Human Skin Fibroblasts Ex Vivo *Diabetes* 53(5): pp 1344-1351

[154]   Ramis, M.R., et al. 2015 Caloric Restriction, Resveratrol and Melatonin: Role of Sirt1 and Implications for Aging and Related-Diseases *Mechanisms of Ageing and Development* 146: pp 28-41

[155]   Armanios, M. 2013 Telomeres and Age-Related Disease: How Telomere Biology Informs Clinical Paradigms *The Journal of Clinical Investigation* 123(3): pp 996-1002

[156]   Van Deursen, J.M. 2014 The Role of Senescent Cells in Ageing *Nature* 509(7501): pp 439

[157]   Shammas, M.A. 2011 Telomeres, Lifestyle, Cancer, and Aging *Current Opinion in Clinical Nutrition and Metabolic Care* 14(1): pp 28

[158]   López-Otín, C., et al. 2013 The Hallmarks of Aging *Cell* 153(6): pp 1194-1217

[159]   Khalangot, M., D. Krasnienkov, and A. Vaiserman 2020 Telomere Length in Different Metabolic Categories: Clinical Associations and Modification Potential *Experimental Biology and Medicine* 245(13): pp 1115-1121

[160]   Al-Thuwaini, T.M. 2021 Association of Antidiabetic Therapy with Shortened Telomere Length in Middle-Aged Type 2 Diabetic Patients *Journal of Diabetes & Metabolic Disorders* 20(2): pp 1161-1168

[161]   Zhang, X., et al. 1999 Telomere Shortening and Apoptosis in Telomerase-Inhibited Human Tumor Cells *Genes and Development* 13(18): pp 2388-2399

[162]   Okuda, K., et al. 2002 Telomere Length in the Newborn *Pediatric Research* 52(3): pp 377-381

[163]   Cawthon, R.M., et al. 2003 Association between Telomere Length in Blood and Mortality in People Aged 60 Years or Older *The Lancet* 361(9355): pp 393-395

[164]   Shin, D., J. Shin, and K.W. Lee 2019 Effects of Inflammation and Depression on Telomere Length in Young Adults in the United States *Journal of Clinical Medicine* 8(5): pp 711

[165]   Sahin, E., et al. 2011 Telomere Dysfunction Induces Metabolic and Mitochondrial Compromise *Nature* 470(7334): pp 359

[166]   Weindruch, R. and R.S. Sohal 1997 Caloric Intake and Aging *New England Journal of Medicine* 337(14): pp 986-994

[167]   Corbyn, Z. 2018 *Want to Live for Ever? Flush out Your Zombie Cells* The Guardian

[168]   Fania, L., et al. 2019 Role of Nicotinamide in Genomic Stability and Skin Cancer Chemoprevention *International Journal of Molecular Sciences* 20(23): pp 5946

[169]   Martínez, D.E. 1998 Mortality Patterns Suggest Lack of Senescence in Hydra *Experimental Gerontology* 33(3): pp 217-225

[170]   Feldscher, K. *In Pursuit of Healthy Aging.* 2017; Available from: https://news.harvard.edu/gazette/story/2017/11/intermittent-fasting-may-be-center-of-increasing-lifespan/.

[171]   Sinclair, D.A. and M.D. LaPlante 2019 *Lifespan: Why We Age—and Why We Don't Have To*: Atria Books

[172]   Fitzgerald, K.N., et al. 2021 Potential Reversal of Epigenetic Age Using a Diet and Lifestyle Intervention: A Pilot Randomized Clinical Trial *Aging* 13(7): pp 9419

[173]   Verdin, E., et al. 2010 Sirtuin Regulation of Mitochondria: Energy Production, Apoptosis, and Signaling *Trends in Biochemical Sciences* 35(12): pp 669-675

[174]   Zhu, Y., et al. 2013 Metabolic Regulation of Sirtuins Upon Fasting and the Implication for Cancer *Current Opinion in Oncology* 25(6): pp 630

[175]   Kanfi, Y., et al. 2008 Regulation of Sirt1 Protein Levels by Nutrient Availability *FEBS Letters* 582(16): pp 2417-2423

[176]   Kane, A.E. and D.A. Sinclair 2018 Sirtuins and Nad+ in the Development and Treatment of Metabolic and Cardiovascular Diseases *Circulation Research* 123(7): pp 868-885

[177]   Kida, Y. and M.S. Goligorsky 2016 Sirtuins, Cell Senescence, and Vascular Aging *Canadian Journal of Cardiology* 32(5): pp 634-641

[178]   Lee, S.-H., et al. 2019 Sirtuin Signaling in Cellular Senescence and Aging *BMB Reports* 52(1): pp 24

[179]   Kincaid, B. and E. Bossy-Wetzel 2013 Forever Young: Sirt3 a Shield against Mitochondrial Meltdown, Aging, and Neurodegeneration *Frontiers in Aging Neuroscience* 5: pp 48

[180]   Hirschey, M.D., et al. 2010 Sirt3 Regulates Mitochondrial Fatty-Acid Oxidation by Reversible Enzyme Deacetylation *Nature* 464(7285): pp 121-125

[181]   Grootaert, M.O., et al. 2021 Sirt6 Protects Smooth Muscle Cells from Senescence and Reduces Atherosclerosis *Circulation research* 128(4): pp 474-491

[182]   Kanfi, Y., et al. 2008 Regulation of Sirt6 Protein Levels by Nutrient Availability *FEBS Letters* 582(5): pp 543-548

[183]   Roichman, A., et al. 2021 Restoration of Energy Homeostasis by Sirt6 Extends Healthy Lifespan *Nature Communications* 12(1): pp 1-18

[184]   Tian, X., et al. 2019 Sirt6 Is Responsible for More Efficient DNA Double-Strand Break Repair in Long-Lived Species *Cell* 177(3): pp 622-638. e22

[185]   Huang, Z., et al. 2018 Identification of a Cellularly Active Sirt6 Allosteric Activator *Nature Chemical Biology* 14(12): pp 1118-1126

[186]   Anderson, K.A., et al. 2017 Metabolic Control by Sirtuins and Other Enzymes That Sense Nad+, Nadh, or Their Ratio *Biochimica et Biophysica Acta (BBA)-Bioenergetics* 1858(12): pp 991-998

[187]   Mehmel, M., N. Jovanović, and U. Spitz 2020 Nicotinamide Riboside—the Current State of Research and Therapeutic Uses *Nutrients* 12(6): pp 1616

[188]   Lautrup, S., et al. 2019 Nad+ in Brain Aging and Neurodegenerative Disorders *Cell Metabolism* 30(4): pp 630-655

[189]   Poljsak, B., V. Kovač, and I. Milisav 2020 Healthy Lifestyle Recommendations: Do the Beneficial Effects Originate from Nad+ Amount at the Cellular Level? *Oxidative Medicine and Cellular Longevity* 2020

[190]   Pirinen, E., et al. 2020 Niacin Cures Systemic Nad+ Deficiency and Improves Muscle Performance in Adult-Onset Mitochondrial Myopathy *Cell Metabolism* 31(6): pp 1078-1090. e5

[191]   de Guia, R.M., et al. 2019 Aerobic and Resistance Exercise Training Reverses Age-Dependent Decline in Nad+ Salvage Capacity in Human Skeletal Muscle *Physiological Reports* 7(12): pp e14139

[192]   Gensous, N., et al. 2020 One-Year Mediterranean Diet Promotes Epigenetic Rejuvenation with Country-and Sex-Specific Effects: A Pilot Study from the Nu-Age Project *Geroscience* 42(2): pp 687-701

[193]   Takahashi, K. and S. Yamanaka 2006 Induction of Pluripotent Stem Cells from Mouse Embryonic and Adult Fibroblast Cultures by Defined Factors *Cell* 126(4): pp 663-676

[194]   Conboy, I.M., et al. 2005 Rejuvenation of Aged Progenitor Cells by Exposure to a Young Systemic Environment *Nature* 433(7027): pp 760

[195]   Regalado, A. *Blood from Old Mice Makes Young Mice Decrepit.* 2016; Available from: https://www.technologyreview.com/s/602897/blood-from-old-mice-makes-young-mice-decrepit/.

[196]   WideCells 2018 How Umbilical Cord Tissue Stem Cell Treatment Helped Mel Gibson's Father Regain a New 'Lease of Life' at 92 *WideCells*

[197]   Iwakiri, R., et al. 2001 Programmed Cell Death in Rat Intestine: Effect of Feeding and Fasting *Scandinavian Journal of Gastroenterology* 36(1): pp 39-47

[198]   Tajes, M., et al. 2010 Neuroprotective Role of Intermittent Fasting in Senescence-Accelerated Mice P8 (Samp8) *Experimental Gerontology* 45(9): pp 702-710

[199]   Sogawa, H. and C. Kubo 2000 Influence of Short-Term Repeated Fasting on the Longevity of Female (Nzb× Nzw) F1 Mice *Mechanisms of Ageing and Development* 115(1-2): pp 61-71

[200]   Goodrick, C., et al. 1990 Effects of Intermittent Feeding Upon Body Weight and Lifespan in Inbred Mice: Interaction of Genotype and Age *Mechanisms of Ageing and Development* 55(1): pp 69-87

[201]   Azzu, V. and T.G. Valencak 2017 Energy Metabolism and Ageing in the Mouse: A Mini-Review *Gerontology* 63(4): pp 327-336

[202]   Fontana, L., L. Partridge, and V.D. Longo 2010 Dietary Restriction, Growth Factors and Aging: From Yeast to Humans *Science* 328(5976): pp 321-326

[203]   Goodrick, C.L., et al. 1983 Differential Effects of Intermittent Feeding and Voluntary Exercise on Body Weight and Lifespan in Adult Rats *Journal of Gerontology* 38(1): pp 36-45

[204]   McCay, C.M., M.F. Crowell, and L.A. Maynard 1935 The Effect of Retarded Growth Upon the Length of Life Span and Upon the Ultimate Body Size: One Figure *The Journal of Nutrition* 10(1): pp 63-79

[205]   Gehrig Jr, J.J., J. Ross, and R.L. Jamison 1988 Effect of Long-Term, Alternate Day Feeding on Renal Function in Aging Conscious Rats *Kidney International* 34(5): pp 620-630

[206]   Tikoo, K., et al. 2007 Intermittent Fasting Prevents the Progression of Type I Diabetic Nephropathy in Rats and Changes the Expression of Sir2 and P53 *FEBS Letters* 581(5): pp 1071-1078

[207]   Han, Y.-m., et al. 2018 B-Hydroxybutyrate Prevents Vascular Senescence through Hnrnp A1-Mediated Upregulation of Oct4 *Molecular Cell* 71(6): pp 1064-1078. e5

[208]   Honjoh, S., et al. 2009 Signalling through Rheb-1 Mediates Intermittent Fasting-Induced Longevity in C. Elegans *Nature* 457(7230): pp 726

[209]   Weir, H.J., et al. 2017 Dietary Restriction and Ampk Increase Lifespan Via Mitochondrial Network and Peroxisome Remodeling *Cell Metabolism* 26(6): pp 884-896. e5

[210]   Yousef, H., et al. 2019 Aged Blood Impairs Hippocampal Neural Precursor Activity and Activates Microglia Via Brain Endothelial Cell Vcam1 *Nature Medicine*: pp 1

[211]   Sanders, N.K. *The Epic of Gilgamesh*. Available from: http://www.aina.org/books.html.

[212]   Fahy, G.M., et al. 2019 Reversal of Epigenetic Aging and Immunosenescent Trends in Humans *Aging Cell* 18(6): pp e13028

[213] Beevers, C.S., et al. 2006 Curcumin Inhibits the Mammalian Target of Rapamycin-Mediated Signaling Pathways in Cancer Cells *International Journal of Cancer* 119(4): pp 757-764

[214] Gomes, A.P., et al. 2013 Declining Nad+ Induces a Pseudohypoxic State Disrupting Nuclear-Mitochondrial Communication During Aging *Cell* 155(7): pp 1624-1638

[215] Houtkooper, R.H. and J. Auwerx 2012 *Exploring the Therapeutic Space around Nad+* Journal of Cell Biology pp 205-209

[216] Fang, E.F., et al. 2016 Nad+ Replenishment Improves Lifespan and Healthspan in Ataxia Telangiectasia Models Via Mitophagy and DNA Repair *Cell Metabolism* 24(4): pp 566-581

[217] Dai, H., et al. 2018 Sirtuin Activators and Inhibitors: Promises, Achievements, and Challenges *Pharmacology & Therapeutics* 188: pp 140-154

[218] Manasa, M., et al. 2012 A Review on Hyaluronic Acid *International Journal of Research in Chemistry and Environment* 2(6)

[219] Capelli, G. and G. Cysewski 2013 *The Worlds' Best Kept Health Secret Natural Astaxanthin*: Kailua-Kona, HI: Cyanotech Corporation

[220] Tobeiha, M., et al. 2022 Evidence for the Benefits of Melatonin in Cardiovascular Disease *Frontiers in Cardiovascular Medicine* 9

[221] Jung-Hynes, B., R.J. Reiter, and N. Ahmad 2010 Sirtuins, Melatonin and Circadian Rhythms: Building a Bridge between Aging and Cancer *Journal of Pineal Research* 48(1): pp 9-19

[222] Gunnars, K. *Grass-Fed Vs. Grain-Fed Beef - What's the Difference?* 2018; Available from: https://www.healthline.com/nutrition/grass-fed-vs-grain-fed-beef.

[223] Ames, B.N., M. Profet, and L.S. Gold 1990 Dietary Pesticides (99.99% All Natural) *Proceedings of the National Academy of Sciences* 87(19): pp 7777-7781

[224] Boffetta, P., et al. 2010 Fruit and Vegetable Intake and Overall Cancer Risk in the European Prospective Investigation into Cancer and Nutrition (Epic) *Journal of the National Cancer Institute* 102(8): pp 529-537

[225] Gunnars, K. *Why Modern Wheat Is Worse Than Older Wheat.* 2014; Available from: https://www.healthline.com/nutrition/modern-wheat-health-nightmare.

[226] Holt, S., J. Miller, and P. Petocz 1997 An Insulin Index of Foods: The Insulin Demand Generated by 1000-Kj Portions of Common Foods *The American Journal of Clinical Nutrition* 66(5): pp 1264-1276

[227] Fothergill, E., et al. 2016 Persistent Metabolic Adaptation 6 Years after "the Biggest Loser" Competition *Obesity* 24(8): pp 1612-1619

[228] Smith, M.W. *Why Am I Losing My Hair?* 2017; Available from: https://www.webmd.com/skin-problems-and-treatments/hair-loss/men-hair-loss-17/male-pattern-baldness.

[229] Hadland, S.E. and S. Levy 2016 Objective Testing: Urine and Other Drug Tests *Child and Adolescent Psychiatric Clinics* 25(3): pp 549-565

[230]   Joseph, P.G. 2012 Serotonergic and Tryptaminergic Overstimulation on Refeeding Implicated in "Enlightenment" Experiences *Medical Hypotheses* 79(5): pp 598-601

[231]   Hazzard, L. 1908 *Fasting for the Cure of Disease* New York City: Physical Culture Publishing Company

[232]   Hazzard, L. 1927 *Scientific Fasting: The Ancient and Modern Key to Health* New York City: Grant Publications Inc

[233]   Shea, M. *Why No One Does Juice Cleanses Anymore*. 2018; Available from: https://nypost.com/2018/01/09/why-no-one-does-juice-cleanses-anymore/.

[234]   Donatelli, J. *The 5 Stages of a Juice Fast*. 2017; Available from: https://www.livestrong.com/article/1011724-s-dr-ozs-3day-detox-cleanse-right-you/.

[235]   Boschmann, M., et al. 2003 Water-Induced Thermogenesis *The Journal of Clinical Endocrinology & Metabolism* 88(12): pp 6015-6019

[236]   Solianik, R., et al. 2016 Effect of 48h Fasting on Autonomic Function, Brain Activity, Cognition, and Mood in Amateur Weight Lifters *BioMed Research International* 2016: pp 1-8

[237]   Frecka, J.M. and R.D. Mattes 2008 Possible Entrainment of Ghrelin to Habitual Meal Patterns in Humans *American Journal of Physiology-Gastrointestinal and Liver Physiology* 294(3): pp G699-G707

[238]   Johnstone, A., et al. 2002 Effect of an Acute Fast on Energy Compensation and Feeding Behaviour in Lean Men and Women *International Journal of Obesity* 26(12): pp 1623

[239]   Choi, I.Y., et al. 2016 A Diet Mimicking Fasting Promotes Regeneration and Reduces Autoimmunity and Multiple Sclerosis Symptoms *Cell Reports* 15(10): pp 2136-2146

[240]   Papagiannopoulos, I.A., et al. 2013 Anthropometric, Hemodynamic, Metabolic, and Renal Responses During 5 Days of Food and Water Deprivation *Complementary Medicine Research* 20(6): pp 427-433

[241]   Kwon, H.M. 2008 Protein Misfolding in Hypertonic Stress: New Insights into an Old Idea. Focus on "Genome-Wide Rnai Screen and in Vivo Protein Aggregation Reporters Identify Degradation of Damaged Protein as an Essential Hypertonic Stress Response" *American Journal of Physiology-Cell Physiology* 295(6): pp C1474-C1475

[242]   Gustin, A. *Dry Fasting: The Truth About This New Health Industry Trend*. 2018; Available from: https://perfectketo.com/dry-fasting/.

[243]   Meckel, Y., A. Ismaeel, and A. Eliakim 2008 The Effect of the Ramadan Fast on Physical Performance and Dietary Habits in Adolescent Soccer Players *European Journal of Applied Physiology* 102(6): pp 651-657

[244]   Davis, C.P. *Dehydration (Adults)*. 2018; Available from: https://www.emedicinehealth.com/heat_stroke/article_em.htm#what_is_the_prognosis_for_heat_stroke.

[245] Adawi, M., et al. 2017 Ramadan Fasting Exerts Immunomodulatory Effects: Insights from a Systematic Review *Frontiers in Immunology*: pp 1144

[246] Longo, V.D., et al. 2021 Intermittent and Periodic Fasting, Longevity and Disease *Nature Aging* 1(1): pp 47-59

[247] Tey, S., et al. 2017 Effects of Aspartame-, Monk Fruit-, Stevia-and Sucrose-Sweetened Beverages on Postprandial Glucose, Insulin and Energy Intake *International Journal of Obesity* 41(3): pp 450

[248] Agricultural Research Service 2018 *Usda Food Composition Databases* United States Department of Agriculture Editor

[249] Caffeine Informer. *20+ Good Health Reasons to Drink Coffee.* 2018; Available from: https://www.caffeineinformer.com/7-good-reasons-to-drink-coffee.

[250] Van Dam, R.M. and E.J. Feskens 2002 Coffee Consumption and Risk of Type 2 Diabetes Mellitus *The Lancet* 360(9344): pp 1477-1478

[251] Cerniuc, C., et al. 2019 Impact of Intermittent Fasting (5: 2) on Ketone Body Production in Healthy Female Subjects *Ernahrungs Umschau* 66(1): pp 2-9

[252] West, H. *How Artificial Sweeteners Affect Blood Sugar and Insulin.* 2017; Available from: https://www.healthline.com/nutrition/artificial-sweeteners-blood-sugar-insulin#section1.

[253] Tea People. *Types of Tea.* 2013; Available from: https://www.teapeople.co.uk/types-of-tea.

[254] Cox, L. *Spirulina: Nutrition Facts & Health Benefits.* 2018; Available from: https://www.livescience.com/48853-spirulina-supplement-facts.html.

[255] Targher, G., et al. 1997 Cigarette Smoking and Insulin Resistance in Patients with Noninsulin-Dependent Diabetes Mellitus *The Journal of Clinical Endocrinology & Metabolism* 82(11): pp 3619-3624

[256] Kubala, J. *The Keto Flu: Symptoms and How to Get Rid of It.* 2018; Available from: https://www.healthline.com/nutrition/keto-flu-symptoms.

[257] Calorie King. *Food Search.* 2018; Available from: https://www.calorieking.com/foods/.

[258] LaFountain, R.A., et al. 2019 Extended Ketogenic Diet and Physical Training Intervention in Military Personnel *Military Medicine*

[259] Nelson, G.J., P.C. Schmidt, and D.S. Kelley 1995 Low-Fat Diets Do Not Lower Plasma Cholesterol Levels in Healthy Men Compared to High-Fat Diets with Similar Fatty Acid Composition at Constant Caloric Intake *Lipids* 30(11): pp 969-976

[260] Bray, G.A. 2010 Fructose: Pure, White, and Deadly? Fructose, by Any Other Name, Is a Health Hazard *Journal of Diabetes Science and Technology* 4(4): pp 1003-1007

[261] Dehghan, M., et al. 2017 Associations of Fats and Carbohydrate Intake with Cardiovascular Disease and Mortality in 18 Countries from Five

Continents (Pure): A Prospective Cohort Study *The Lancet* 390(10107): pp 2050-2062

[262]   Elamin, M., et al. 2017 Ketone-Based Metabolic Therapy: Is Increased Nad+ a Primary Mechanism? *Frontiers in Molecular Neuroscience* 10: pp 377

[263]   Youm, Y.-H., et al. 2015 The Ketone Metabolite B-Hydroxybutyrate Blocks Nlrp3 Inflammasome–Mediated Inflammatory Disease *Nature Medicine* 21(3): pp 263-269

[264]   Ji, C., et al. 2020 A Ketogenic Diet Attenuates Proliferation and Stemness of Glioma Stemlike Cells by Altering Metabolism Resulting in Increased Ros Production *International Journal of Oncology* 56(2): pp 606-617

[265]   Loria, K. *A Strange Diet Is Designed to Slow Aging by Mimicking Fasting - Here's How It Works and What People Eat.* 2018; Available from: https://www.businessinsider.my/valter-longo-prolon-fasting-diet-cost-does-it-work-2018-4/?r=US&IR=T.

[266]   Brandhorst, S., et al. 2015 A Periodic Diet That Mimics Fasting Promotes Multi-System Regeneration, Enhanced Cognitive Performance, and Healthspan *Cell Metabolism* 22(1): pp 86-99

[267]   Mowll, B. *What Is the Fasting Mimicking Diet?* 2018; Available from: https://drmowll.com/what-is-the-fasting-mimicking-diet/.

[268]   Kim, J. *Intermittent Fasting: The Complete Guide.* 2016; Available from: http://hackyour.fitness/intermittent-fasting-complete-guide/.

[269]   Robinson, C. *Getting Started.* Available from: https://www.snakediet.com/getting-started/.

[270]   Biswas, C. *The One Meal a Day Diet (Omad Diet) – How It Works, Health Benefits, and Safety.* 2018; Available from: https://www.stylecraze.com/articles/one-meal-a-day-diet-the-ultimate-guide/#gref.

[271]   Horton, B. *Intermittent Fasting Made Easy.* 2018; Available from: https://theblakediet.com/.

[272]   Bray, G.A. 2004 Medical Consequences of Obesity *The Journal of Clinical Endocrinology & Metabolism* 89(6): pp 2583-2589

[273]   Redman, L.M. and E. Ravussin 2011 Caloric Restriction in Humans: Impact on Physiological, Psychological, and Behavioral Outcomes *Antioxidants & Redox Signaling* 14(2): pp 275-287

[274]   Fildes, A., et al. 2015 Probability of an Obese Person Attaining Normal Body Weight: Cohort Study Using Electronic Health Records *American Journal of Public Health* 105(9): pp e54-e59

[275]   National Center for Health Statistics. *Prevalence of Overweight, Obesity, and Severe Obesity among Adults Aged 20 and Over: United States, 1960–1962 through 2015–2016.* 2018; Available from: https://www.cdc.gov/nchs/data/hestat/obesity_adult_15_16/obesity_adult_15_16.htm.

[276]   Brillat-Savarin, J.A. 1825 The Physiology of Taste: Or Meditations on Transcendental Gastronomy, Trans *MFK Fisher, New York, Everyman's Library*

[277]   Centers for Disease Control and Prevention 2018 *Nutrition, Physical Activity, and Obesity: Data, Trends and Maps*

[278]   Yudkin, J. 1986 *Pure, White and Deadly*: Penguin Random House UK

[279]   Bellisle, F., R. McDevitt, and A.M. Prentice 1997 Meal Frequency and Energy Balance *British Journal of Nutrition* 77(S1): pp S57-S70

[280]   Verboeket-Van De Venne, W.P., K.R. Westerterp, and A.D. Kester 1993 Effect of the Pattern of Food Intake on Human Energy Metabolism *British Journal of Nutrition* 70(1): pp 103-115

[281]   Tremaroli, V. and F. Bäckhed 2012 Functional Interactions between the Gut Mcrobiota and Hst Mtabolism *Nature* 489(7415): pp 242

[282]   Clemente, J.C., et al. 2012 The Impact of the Gut Microbiota on Human Health: An Integrative View *Cell* 148(6): pp 1258-1270

[283]   Varady, K. 2011 Intermittent Versus Daily Calorie Restriction: Which Diet Regimen Is More Effective for Weight Loss? *Obesity Reviews* 12(7): pp e593-e601

[284]   Gunnars, K. *Protein Intake – How Much Protein Should You Eat Per Day?* 2018; Available from: https://www.healthline.com/nutrition/how-much-protein-per-day.

[285]   Harvard Health Publishing 2009 *Listing of Vitamins* H.M. School Editor

[286]   Del Corral, P., et al. 2009 Effect of Dietary Adherence with or without Exercise on Weight Loss: A Mechanistic Approach to a Global Problem *The Journal of Clinical Endocrinology & Metabolism* 94(5): pp 1602-1607

[287]   Segal, B. *Heart Attacks at 50 Years Old.* 2016; Available from: https://www.focusforhealth.org/heart-attacks-at-50-years-old/.

[288]   Dixon, J.B., et al. 2008 Adjustable Gastric Banding and Conventional Therapy for Type 2 Diabetes: A Randomized Controlled Trial *Jama* 299(3): pp 316-323

[289]   Das, S.K., et al. 2003 Long-Term Changes in Energy Expenditure and Body Composition after Massive Weight Loss Induced by Gastric Bypass Surgery *The American Journal of Clinical Nutrition* 78(1): pp 22-30

[290]   Lingvay, I., et al. 2013 Rapid Improvement of Diabetes after Gastric Bypass Surgery: Is It the Diet or Surgery? *Diabetes Care*: pp DC_122316

[291]   Web MD. *Paying for Weight Loss Surgery.* 2018; Available from: https://www.webmd.com/diet/obesity/financing-weight-loss-surgery#1.

[292]   CostHelper. *Heart Bypass Surgery Cost.* 2018.

[293]   Bean, M. *10 Most Popular Prescription Drugs for 2017.* 2017; Available from: https://www.beckershospitalreview.com/supply-chain/10-most-popular-prescription-drugs-for-2017.html.

[294]   Media Relations. *New Cdc Report: More Than 100 Million Americans Have Diabetes or Prediabetes.* 2017; Available from: https://www.cdc.gov/media/releases/2017/p0718-diabetes-report.html.

[295]   Konish, L. *You May Want to Rethink This Strategy for Claiming Social Security Early.* 2018; Available from: https://www.cnbc.com/2018/04/06/you-may-want-to-rethink-this-strategy-for-claiming-social-security-early.html.

[296]   Munro, D. *U.S. Healthcare Hits $3 Trillion.* 2012; Available from: https://www.forbes.com/sites/danmunro/2012/01/19/u-s-healthcare-hits-3-trillion/#3d1457023da8.

[297]   O'Callaghan, T. *Why Are Foreigners Coming to Russia to Starve Themselves?* ; Available from: https://www.rbth.com/lifestyle/327016-foreigners-coming-to-starve-themselves.

[298]   Lieberman, H.R., et al. 2008 A Double-Blind, Placebo-Controlled Test of 2 D of Calorie Deprivation: Effects on Cognition, Activity, Sleep, and Interstitial Glucose Concentrations *The American Journal of Clinical Nutrition* 88(3): pp 667-676

[299]   Woodfield, J. *The Story of Angus Barbieri, Who Went 382 Days without Eating.* 2018; Available from: https://www.diabetes.co.uk/blog/2018/02/story-angus-barbieri-went-382-days-without-eating/.

[300]   Stewart, W. and L.W. Fleming 1973 Features of a Successful Therapeutic Fast of 382 Days' Duration *Postgraduate Medical Journal* 49(569): pp 203-209

[301]   Medical Bag. *The Origins of Soda.* 2014; Available from: https://www.medicalbag.com/grey-matter/the-origins-of-soda/article/472378/.

I was born in a small town in Michigan, filled with the noises of factories. While growing up, I witnessed factory closures, which brought high unemployment and few economic opportunities. I left the town to pursue my dreams and enrolled in a university. My education opened the door to the world, where I graduated with a Ph.D. in environmental and natural resource economics from Texas A&M University. With my degree, I traveled and lived in Bosnia and Herzegovina, the Republic of Kazakhstan, Morocco, Malaysia, and the United States. Currently, I teach economics and finance at a small university in Morocco. Despite my humble beginnings as a poor boy from Michigan, I am doing alright. I am living life to the fullest.

Other books from the author:

The Arduous Path to Enlightenment

As human beings, we often ponder upon our existence on this earth and ask ourselves why we are here. We search for answers through various religions like Hinduism, Buddhism, Christianity, Islam, and Judaism. They share a common theme where God wants us to use all our talents and become closer to Him. We examine methods like fasting, meditation, lucid dreaming, sensory deprivation, and mind-altering drugs such as psychedelics and marijuana to explore our minds and awaken our spirituality. We delve into the deep depths of our minds and psyches to gain greater awareness and uncover hidden aspects of ourselves. Through this journey, we discover our true selves and purpose in life while traversing the path to enlightenment.

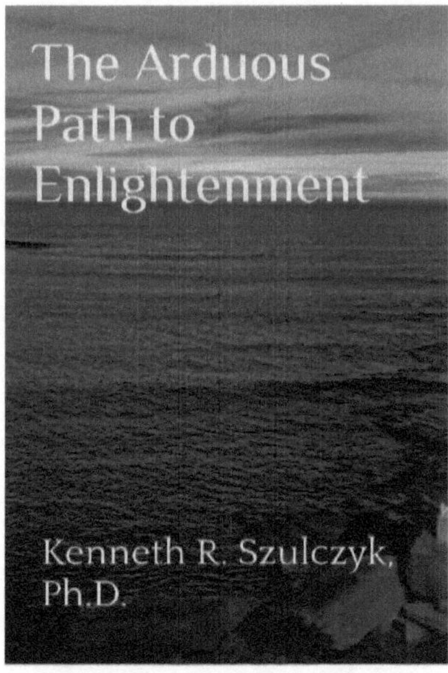

The Rise of the Insane State - What is Happening…

This book offers a comprehensive view of the U.S. legal system, explaining the relationships between the people, businesses, and their government. It is not filled with complicated statistics or high-level economic jargon. It is written for any intelligent person who wants to understand why a government takes over its economy. The book uses numerous examples and cases from the United States, but these ideas can apply to any country. It is a book that makes complex concepts accessible and understandable.

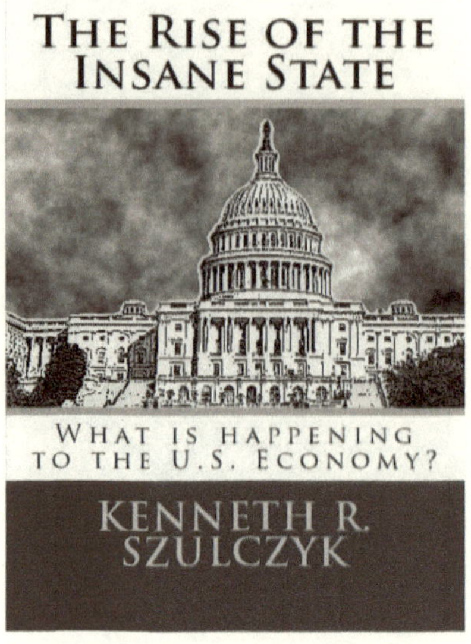

Paying for College – The Novel

Brothers, I only wanted to attend a university and escape a small town with no job prospects or future. But every time I opened my mailbox at the dorm, I pulled out another tuition bill with a looming due date. So, I had to do the unthinkable—break a few rules and do some insane things. Then everything just became crazy.

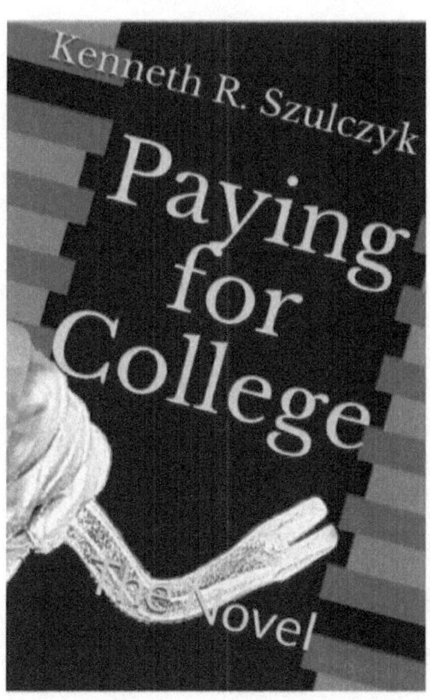

To Tame Man

The United Federation of Cities has been at peace since the Great War, and one of its great cities, Chicago, has experienced no violence, no crime, and no murders in 68 years. Then Susan, the director of the Male Processing Unit, ran out of Growth Inhibitor 37, and several males, including Brown 447, did not get their treatment. Unfortunately, Brown 447 shows an uncanny intelligence and rises up and challenges the society of Chicago. Mayor Lilith and the Mayor's Guards must restore the social order and return law and order to Chicago.

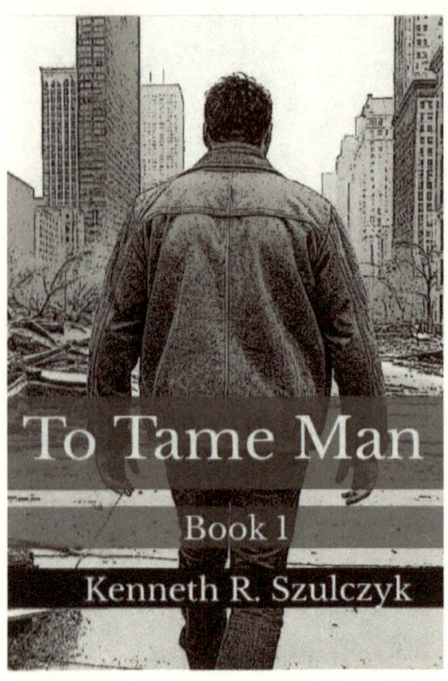

Searching for Stolen Love

Fox is an American finance professor. He is thrilled to teach at the Bosnian University of Management, a place, where he hopes to make a difference. His future is bright, and he fell in love with a Serbian woman. Having just completed his first semester, he is looking forward to a peaceful winter. But one night, his girlfriend disappeared without a trace, and he is left with a growing sense of unease. Determined to find her, Fox embarks on a search that would lead him to uncover a mystery in the land of blood and honey.

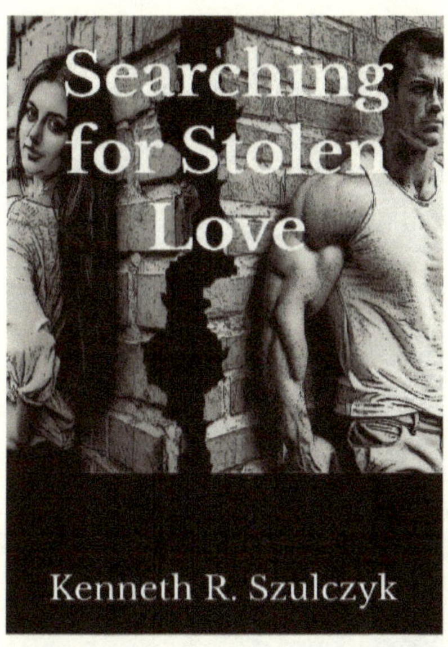

The Second American Revolution - The Building...

As a child, Jerrick Ray Davis dreamed of delivering powerful speeches to the people. He also dreams of building an Empire across the North and South Americas. These are not simple daydreams but ideas that map out Jerrick's destiny. Jerrick rises out of the wreckage and devastation of the Michigan economy and turns his dreams into reality. Jerrick Davis and his political party, the National Workers' Party, took over the United States government and the rest of the Americas. Jerrick Ray Davis becomes the most powerful man in the 21st century, and the world trembles at his sight. Jerrick Ray Davis also makes a promise to the people. After the 2008 Financial Crisis, he will put all Americans back to work. Good-paying jobs will be plentiful again. Of course, Jerrick Davis puts everyone back to work, building his Empire. This story is about Jerrick Ray Davis' life from early childhood to rising in power. Please read this story with caution; we may be all toiling hard on Jerrick Ray Davis' Empire. As Jerrick Ray Davis says, "All Americans will be united under one flag."

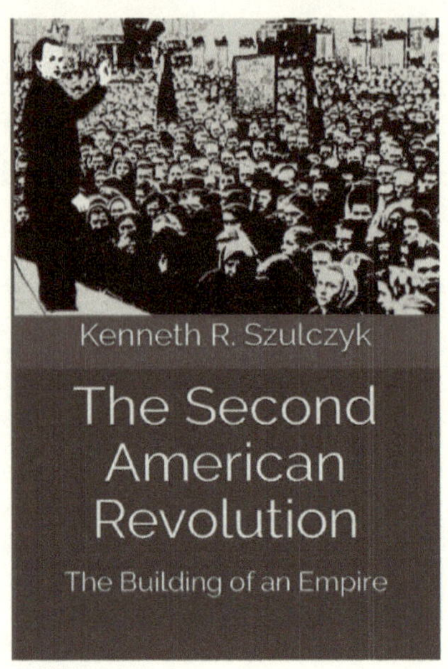
Kenneth R. Szulczyk
The Second
American
Revolution
The Building of an Empire

9 781790 787586